MEDICAL RADIOLOGY

Diagnostic Imaging and Radiation Oncology

Practical Approaches to Cancer Invasion and Metastases

A Compendium of Radiation Oncologists' Responses to 40 Histories

Contributors

B.S. Aron · S.O. Asbell · J.A. Battle · J.M. Bedwinek · W.A. Bethune · L.W. Brady
T.J. Brickner · T.A. Buchholz · J.R. Cassady · J.R. Castro · C.M. Chahbazian
J.S. Cooper · R.R. Dobelbower, Jr. · R.W. Edland · A.M. El-Mahdi · A.L. Goldson
H. Goepfert · T.W. Griffin · S. Gupta · E.C. Halperin · J.C. Hernandez · D.H. Hussey
N. Kaufman · H.D. Kerman · H.M. Keys · C.M. Mansfield · J.E. Marks
S.A. Marks · B. Micaily · M.J. Miller · W.T. Moss · K. Murray · L.J. Peters
R.D. Pezner · L.R. Prosnitz · M. Raben · H. Reiter · T.A. Rich · P. Rubin
M.C. Ryoo · R.H. Sagerman · O.M. Salazar · R.K. Schmidt-Ulrich · C.L. Shields
J.A. Shields · B.L. Speiser · A.D. Steinfeld · M. Suntharalingam · M.A. Tomé
D.Y. Tong · J. Tsao · J.F. Wilson

Edited by A. Robert Kagan

With the Assistance of Richard J. Steckel

Foreword by

Luther W. Brady and H.-P. Heilmann

Springer-Verlag
Berlin Heidelberg New York
London Paris Tokyo
Hong Kong Barcelona
Budapest

A. Robert Kagan, MD

Southern California Permanente Medical Group
Department of Radiation Oncology
4950 Sunset Boulevard 2C
Los Angeles, CA 90027
USA

Richard J. Steckel, MD

University of California, Los Angeles
Center for Health Sciences
Johnsson Cancer Center
10833 Le Conte
Los Angeles, CA 90024
USA

MEDICAL RADIOLOGY · Diagnostic Imaging and Radiation Oncology

Continuation of
Handbuch der medizinischen Radiologie
Encyclopedia of Medical Radiology

With 7 Figures and 2 Tables

ISBN-13: 978-3-642-84887-2 e-ISBN-13: 978-3-642-84885-8
DOI: 10.1007/978-3-642-84885-8

Library of Congress Cataloging-in-Publication Data
Practical approaches to cancer invasion and metastases : a compendium of radiation oncologists' responses to 40 histories/ with contributions by B.S. Aron.... [et. al.] ; edited by A. Robert Kagan with the assistance of Richard J. Steckel ; foreword by Luther W. Brady and H.-P. Heilmann. p. cm. — (Medical radiology) Includes bibliographical references and index.

1. Metastasis — Case studies. 2. Cancer invasiveness — Case studies. 3. Cancer — Radiotherapy — Case studies. I. Aron, Bernard S. II. Kagan.
A. Robert (Arthur Robert). 1936-. III. Steckel, Richard J., 1936-. IV. Series. [DNLM:1.Neoplasm Invasiveness — case studies. 2. Neoplasm Metastasis is — case studies. Qz 202 P895 1994] RC269.5.P73 1994 616.99407 — dc20 DNLM/DLC for Library of Congress 93-42006

Softcover reprint of the hardcover 1st edition 1994

Typesetting: Thomson Press (I) Ltd, New Delhi
SPIN: 10044454 21/3130/SPS - 5 4 3 2 1 0 - Printed on acid-free paper

Foreword

In the United States in 1993 the American Cancer Society estimated that there were about 1,300,000 new cases of invasive cancer diagnosed. At the time of presentation about 70% of those patients represented limited local regional disease without evidences of distant dissemination. About 30% of the patients had demonstrated metastatic disease at the time of initial diagnosis or about 390,000 patients.

Of those patients with local regional disease about 56% would be cured by the best treatment programs including surgery, radiation therapy with or without chemotherapy when given for cure. Therefore, of the 1,300,000 new cases of invasive cancer, about 509,000 would be cured by the best treatments available.

However, about 790,000 patients will have metastatic disease as a part of initial presentation or following the completion of definitive treatment.

The majority of the patients with metastatic disease will have metastases to bone as the dominant site of metastatic disease primarily from cancers of the breast and lung but other metastatic sites will be common including lung, liver, mediastinal and retro-peritoneal lymph node groups as well as brain and spinal cord. It has been suggested by SMITHERS, CARLING and WINDEYER that the management of the patient with metastatic disease or recurrent disease can be a more difficult problem in management than a patient who is treated for cure. The management of metastatic disease, therefore, tries the expertise, intellectual efforts of all of the physicians managing the patient not only in the decision-making process with regards to the treatment program to be pursued but, also, the development of the treatment program for the patient and its actual execution.

KAGAN and STECKEL in their book, *Practical Approaches to Cancer Invasion and Metastases*, have presented a series of case studies for review, definition of a problem, decision relative to treatment and the definition of the most appropriate treatment program with the evidence documenting the process as well as the evidence supporting the choice of treatments to be pursued.

The book represents a unique and important effort in education with actual case studies to illustrate the important points in the process of development of the treatment program.

The case study technology was first used in the evolution of teaching programs in *Skeletal Radiology*. The authors have continued that exploration in the unique and important approach to the development of treatment programs in metastatic disease. It represents a truly innovative approach to the problem. It will serve as a useful tool not only for students of radiation oncology but, also, for practicing physicians in radiation oncology.

Philadelphia/Hamburg, February 1994

L. W. BRADY
H.-P. HEILMANN

Preface

We are not sure how the notion developed that scientific writings in medicine must adhere to a uniform stylistic pattern. Following a single format in contributions to an edited volume may indeed lead to uniformity, which promotes familiarity but not individuality. Those who are anticipating a single format for the contributions to this book, as in the "best" edited volumes, may be disappointed.

Lewis Thomas said: "Of all the facts of cooperative behavior to be observed anywhere in nature, I can think of nothing to match, for the free exchange of assets and the achievement of equity and balance in the trade, *human language*... it contains the two most characteristic and accommodating of all human traits, ambiguity and amiability. *Almost every message in human communication can be taken in two or more ways*". ... We are obliged to listen more carefully, to edit whatever we hear and to recognize uncertainty when we hear it or *read it*" (editor's emphasis).

Each contributing author to this book has been allowed to choose his own format in describing his approach to a proffered case history from the editors. Case histories were assigned to expert discussants at random. Each expert we approached was asked to request a different case history if, for some reason, the assigned one was unacceptable. Some of the replies that the experts contributed are long, some short, some with many and others with few references. Some contributors have spoken directly to the individual patient's problem(s); other contributors have hedged their recommendations. Some felt uncomfortable with the brevity of the case history we provided; others have interpolated "clinical information" of their own, to add definition to the information provided them by the editors.

Most contributors have been reluctant to suggest a "no specific treatment" option, or a referral to a hospice. To be asked to comment on the management of a patient may oblige an expert consultant to take a "proactive" role; it is worrisome that the recommended management strategy may then be dictated to some extent by the availability of technical means, rather than by the desired clinical ends.

Our current cancer management environment enshrouds us with the vocabulary of warriors or activists: "the war on cancer," "task force committees," and "consensus conferences." Inherent in the precepts about clinical management that are generated by some "establishment" committees and authoritative oncology texts is the notion that the active physician is "good" and the passive physician is "bad," or at least inadequate. Are we as radiation oncologists so transfixed upon our past glories in curing localized cancer of the endolarynx, breast, and cervix with "the beam," that we reflexively turn on the beam also to treat multiple brain metastases, stage IV cancer of the lung, and recurrent epithelial malignancies with similar expectations? Clearly, meditating on the wisdom of *any* treatment or contemplating the best management for cancer patients with large, incurable cancers and widespread metastatic disease needs to be done in a framework that acknowledges the unyielding complexity of some of these problems. Discussions of the management of patients with incurable cancer should also be elevated to the same level of visibility and concern as those of curative treatments.

Each contributing expert to this book has described his personal view, using his own communicative style, of the best management for the patient problem assigned. Some contributors may have received more difficult patient problems than others, but *all* have been good "players" in this exercise of clinical judgement without having personal access to the patient. We, the editors, solicit the comments of you, the readers.

Los Angeles, CA, February 1994

A. ROBERT KAGAN
RICHARD J. STECKEL

Contents

Introduction

Statistical significance has very limited applicability to studies of patients with metastatic disease. A study result may be judged "statistically significant" if it is unlikely to have occurred by chance. However, the result may not mean much for the management of *individual* patients with metastases (DEAN 1986; FEIN 1986; KASSEL 1974). The extent of the metastatic involvement, the severity of the debilitating effects on the patient, the speed of the metastatic process, the presence or absence of visceral metastases, and the patient's Karnofsky (performance) status, in addition to many other factors, make the statistical evaluation of groups of patients of little practical significance. Complex emotional factors may also make the management of individual patients extremely difficult. The oncologist, the patient or the patient's family often want "everything" to be done. Because of their perceived importance in the minds of many dying patients, oncologists themselves may sometimes indulge in magical thinking, searching for the miracle of "medicine X" which may be better than nothing (but not by much). Careful consideration of the critical trade-offs, which is so necessary in decision-making for patients with metastases, may be interpreted as therapeutic nihilism. Trade-offs between possible benefits of treatments and their price and between therapy-induced toxicity and the maintenance of normal life-style, are frequently muddled or forgotten, and this lack of clarity adds "costs" for everyone. For example, it is a common practice to employ antineoplastic chemotherapy when the anticipated response rate is 20%; usually survival is not prolonged, quality of life is not maintained, and the cost and time spent in the doctor's office or hospital is excessive (MOERTEL 1991; HOLLI and HAKAMA 1991; MAHER et al. 1990). Patients may also be irradiated again and again while ignoring evidence that radiations are ineffective (MAHER et al. 1990; MAHER 1991).

Asking the patient or the patient's designated agent what he or she wants should be central for determining management. The majority of patients referred to our radiation oncology department have far too many tests and imaging studies which do not contribute to clinical decision making, and we are often told that it is the patient who wants "everything" done! In actuality, we find that no one has asked the patient directly what she or he wants. No one has talked to the family. Worse, the patient may simply be told he will be irradiated and that it will "fix everything." Some patients are so frightened or poorly informed they don't know what they want.

Clinical judgement as documented by the individual discussions in this volume, an important part of which is listening and talking to patients, is the key to decision-making in patients with metastatic disease. There is no "recipe" to define the patient for whom no surgical, radiotherapeutic or chemotherapeutic modality may be effective. In fact, there can be no preset definition of what is effective therapy!

Only a small number of all clinical interventions are proved by objective and incontrovertible evidence to do more good than harm. If we had indisputable evidence that most interventions by oncologists were of clear benefit to patients, there would be no need for this book! In 1981 Couch analyzed surgical errors over a 1-year period at the Peter Bent Brigham Hospital (COUCH et al. 1981). Since 1981 these errors, mostly ones of commission, have persisted in all fields of oncology: misplaced optimism, unwarranted urgency, urge for perfection, and performance of new "stylistic" regimens.

In 1991, Moss wrote "the care of the patient with incurable metastatic cancer makes you lie awake nights wondering if you are doing more harm than good....every patient has so many variables to be balanced in coming to an 'optimum' treatment decision" (W. Moss, personal communication).

Many agree that patients with advanced cancer are often overtreated and overinvestigated to the disadvantage of the patients, their loved ones and society (GOETZLER and MOSKOWITZ 1991). While there is still no universal agreement, some subsets of patients with advanced and incurable disease should probably be excluded from active treatment; for example, patients suffering cardiopulmonary arrest, those needing emergency operations while under palliative chemotherapy, and patients with preterminal prognostic signs such as carcinomatous hypercalcemia (Ferrara et al. 1982; Chevrolet and Jolliet 1991; Blackwell 1987; Vitelli et al. 1991). Unfortunately, medical schools and postgraduate training programs fail to instill humble values and encourage common sense in students and trainees, and focus instead on emerging technologies. It is a sad fact that oncologists in a fee-for-service environment may never look at these issues seriously until such time as resources are truly limited and the economic incentives for maximum treatment are eliminated.

This book is intended to serve as a beginning discussion of the management of patients with metastatic disease by the radiation oncologist. Where do you draw the line for saying "no" to treatment? How does one come to a no-treatment decision? Certainly with a great deal of difficulty, especially after a prior experience with humiliation from a contrary second opinion or even the distant threat of a malpractice suit. No one is taught how to discuss no treatment for cancer with patients or patients' families. In this book we have tried to present some common clinical problems that have caused debate in our department. How do other radiation therapists in the United States discuss and solve these problems?

During the past year we have also surveyed medical oncologists and surgical oncologists, as well as radiation oncologists informally to ascertain how they reach decisions in patients with metastatic disease. While management decisions on these patients must be made daily, no one has yet been able to specify categorical criteria for (1) defining the "preterminal" patient, (2) defining the patient for hospice referral, and (3) defining the patient who is to receive no antineoplastic treatment.

Perhaps it is best to have no consensus on complicated patient management issues, as issues (Skrabanek 1991). This leaves room for imaginative thought and new ideas in the service of each patient. But there is a sufficient body of facts adding up to useful knowledge and sometimes "truth," that can be taught to trainees and shared among seasoned radiation oncologists (Bunting et al. 1992; Rilke 1991; DiFuria et al. 1991).

Bill Rider once said that the practice of curative radiation therapy would almost be "perfect" if you had the luxury of observing the patient for 3 months and irradiating only the patients whose lesions did not grow in that time (B. Rider, personal communication).

Excluding patients with oncologic emergencies, treating the symptoms only and withholding judgement in a severely symptomatic patient for 1 week to observe stability or a rapid downhill course is a tactic often denied by the referring physician, the patient or family members who desire immediate treatment. While there is no scientific definition of a dying patient, the trend in Karnofsky status or neurological status over a short period may serve as the best evaluable parameter for deciding on treatment, even while in practice it is usually difficult to employ.

Another problem we experience in the management of patients with metastatic disease is the expectation of "miracles" and the lack of commitment by oncologists to reverse this impression. Most common is the scenario of the cancer patient who has severe back ache or headache with bone destruction or multiple cerebral masses and who is referred for treatment after a positive imaging study and no substantive discussion with the patient – or, worse, with a discussion that implies the possibility of cure after treatment.

Doubtless, in such instances we may be severely challenged to follow a policy of complete honesty with the patient and/or his family. Being introduced for the first time to a patient with advanced cancer and then trying to do a medical and psychological evaluation may be traumatic to the doctor as well as the patient! At this stage the patient may be so ill or depressed that he is unable to think clearly and say what he wants done. To acknowledge this problem is not to solve it. Furthermore, radiation oncologists get paid for treating patients, not talking to them.

Our impression is that little is known about how we as radiation oncologists manage patients with metastatic disease. How are decisions made? One can read about principles of management but, unlike *curative* radiation therapy where there is some recognizable relationship between principles and practice, we have often failed to see that relationship when the issue is a patient with metastatic disease. Hence the justification for this volume.

References

Blackwell LJ (1987) Must we always use CPR? N Engl J Med 20: 1281–1284

Bunting RV, Boublik M, Blevins FT, Dame CC, Ford LA, Lavine LS (1992) Functional outcome of pathologic fracture secondary to malignant disease in a rehabilitation hospital. Cancer 69: 98–102

Chevrolet JC, Jolliet P (1991) An ethical look at intensive care for patients with malignancies. Eur J Cancer 27: 210–212

Couch NP, Tilney NL, Rayner AA, Moore FD (1981) The high-cost of low-frequency events: the anatomy and economics of surgical mishaps. N Engl J Med 304(11): 634–637
Dean RE (1986) When Jennie took to bed. JAMA 255: 650
DiFuria L, Piga A, Marmili S, Breccia R, Rubini C, Beltrami CA, Mariuzzi GM, Cellerino R (1991) The value of necropsy in oncology. Eur J Cancer 27: 559–561
Fein AR (1986) The state of the art. JAMA 255: 1488
Ferrara JJ, Martin EW Jr, Carey LC (1982) Morbidity of emergency operations in patients with metastatic cancer receiving chemotherapy. Surgery 92: 605–609
Goetzler RM, Moskowitz MA (1991) Changes in physician attitudes toward limiting care of critically ill patients. Arch Intern Med 151: 1537–1540
Holli K, Hakama M (1991) Terminal stages of breast cancer: changes in clinical practice. Eur J Cancer 27: 1338–1339
Kassel V (1974) The penalty for smoking. JAMA 227: 941
Maher EJ (1991) The influence of national attitudes on the use of radiotherapy in advanced and metastatic cancer, with particular reference to differences between the United Kingdom and the United States of America: implications for future studies. Int J Radiat Oncol Biol Phys 20: 1369–1373
Maher EJ, Dische S, Grosch E, Fermont D, Ashford R, Saunders M, Makepeace A, Korn M, Shah D (1990) Who gets radiotherapy? Health Trends 22: 78–83
Moertel CG (1991) Off-label drug use for cancer therapy and national health care priorities. JAMA 266: 3031–3032
Rilke F (1991) The autopsy: its role in oncology. Eur J Cancer 27: 528–530
Skrabanek P (1991) Who needs consensus? Eur J Cancer 27: 523–524
Vitelli CE, Cooper K, Rogatko A, Brennan MF (1991) Cardiopulmonary resuscitation and the patient with cancer. J Clin Oncol 9: 111–115

Part I Prolong Life

It appears to me a most excellent thing for the physician to cultivate Prognosis; for by foreseeing and foretelling, in the presence of the sick, the present, the past, and the future, and explaining the omissions which patients have been guilty of, he will be the more readily believed to be acquainted with the circumstances of the sick; so that men will have confidence to extract themselves to such a physician. And he will manage the cure best who has foreseen what is to happen from the present state of matters.... Thus a man will be the more esteemed to be a good physician, for he will be the better able to treat those aright who can be saved, from having long anticipated everything; and by seeing and announcing beforehand those who will die, he will thus escape censure.

HIPPOCRATES

He who would teach men to die would teach them to live.

MICHEL DE MONTAIGNE

Introduction

There can be little doubt, as major technological advances have occurred, that some patients are kept alive longer than necessary. The difference between prolonging life and prolonging death has become smaller, once the quality of life factor is accounted for. Increasing numbers of invasive procedures are being done on near-dying patients: chest tubes, tracheostomies, feeding gastrostomies (and jejunostomies), central lines, vascular access procedures, diagnostic laparotomies (or endoscopies) for an abdominal complaint, multiple laparotomies for bowel obstruction due to carcinomatosis. Finally, is it not a "sin" for a patient to die at any time from gastrointestinal hemorrhage?

Are there any physicians in educational roles who will put forth, or at least discuss a no-treatment recommendation for the patient with cancer of the lung and brain metastases? Admittedly, pressures often demand that something be done, and it is easier to comply with these than to oppose. How about our responsibility to "do no harm" and to make the patient comfortable?

How can we teach ourselves to say "no," and then be able to convey this message compassionately to patient and family?

Each discussant of the case histories to follow has had to ask himself how energetically to treat: radical early, conservative late – perhaps; radical early, radical late, may be more common.

1 Advanced Rhabdomyosarcoma of the Sinus

E.C. Halperin

One year ago an 18-year-old woman was treated for an alveolar rhabdomyosarcoma (RMS) of the right maxillary sinus which presented with unilateral proptosis and severe facial swelling associated with complete opacification of unilateral sinuses and the sphenoid. Bilateral adenopathy was palpated. A rapid complete remission was obtained after multiagent chemotherapy and then 5000 cGy was delivered to the primary and neck.

Within 9 months after diagnosis, paraplegia occurred associated with a complete block at T7 and a positive cerebrospinal fluid (CSF) cytology.

1. Was this patient potentially curable?
2. Should the entire nervous system have been treated initially?
3. What is the goal now – cure? palliation?
4. When would you recommend hospice?

Response

RMS is a highly malignant neoplasm of striated muscle composed of cells derived from primitive mesenchyme. It represents between 5% and 15% of all malignant solid tumors in patients less than 15 years of age (Bonilla and Healy 1989). RMS includes, but is not limited to, cells with recognizable cross-striations. Cytogenetic analysis has found that many of these tumors have a chromosomal translocation (Anonymous 1989; MacArthur et al. 1992).There are four histologic types of RMS classically described. The *embryonal* form resembles normally developing skeletal muscle in a 7- to 10-week-old fetus while the *alveolar* form resembles the skeletal muscle of the 10- to 20-week-old fetus. A subtype of embryonal RMS is referred to as sarcoma botryoides because of a layer of spindle cells pushing up beneath the mucosa causing polypoid masses resembling a bunch of grapes. *Pleomorphic* RMS has large cells and multinucleated cells mixed with spindle cells and strap cells. The *mixed* RMS contains more than one of the above histologic types within the same tumor (Anderson et al. 1990; Grieman et al. 1988; Salloum et al. 1989). The prognosis of RMS varies as a function of the histologic type. Alveolar RMS generally has a worse prognosis compared to the embryonal, pleomorphic, or mixed variants (Halperin et al.(1989); Salloum et al. 1989).

It is interesting to speculate on the origin of a RMS in the paranasal sinuses of this patient. It has been suggested that such tumors originate either from misplaced embryonic muscle cells or that there is teratomatous growth of heterologous tissues and mesenchymal derivatives into RMS (Grieman et al. 1988).

RMS constituted 22.3% of all malignant tumors of the head and neck seen at St Sophia Children's Hospital of Athens from 1964 to 1983, and 28% of malignant head and neck neoplasms seen in children at the Institut Gustave-Roussy from 1975 to 1987. Thus, RMS vies with non-Hodgkin's lymphoma, Hodgkin's disease, and nasopharyngeal carcinoma as the single most common childhood malignancy presenting in the head and neck (Rapidis et al. 1988; Schwaab et al. 1989).

The common sites of origin of RMS include the orbit (9%), parameningeal sites of the head and neck defined as the middle ear, nasal cavity and paranasal sinuses, nasopharynx, infratemporal fossa/pterygopalatine region, and parapharyngeal areas (18%); other head and neck sites (9%), trunk (7%), and gastrointestinal, perineum/anus, and intrathoracic sites (Crist et al. 1990; Halperin et al. 1989). Primary RMS of the maxillary sinus is rare (Grieman et al. 1988).

The distribution of RMS tumor histology varies by primary site. About 50% of extremity RMS primaries are of alveolar histology and 24% embryonal. This may be compared to orbital lesions where 80% are embryonal and 5% alveolar. At head and neck sites other than the orbit, such as the patient

Edward C. Halperin, MD, Associate Professor, Duke University Medical Center, P.O. Box 3085, Durham, NC 27710, USA

described, about 70% are embryonal histology and 30% alveolar (Crist et al. 1990; Halperin et al. 1989).

For many years there was no universally accepted staging system for RMS. The most commonly used system was the Intergroup Rhabdomyosarcoma (IRS) grouping. This was a surgical-pathologic system where group 1 referred to localized disease which was completely resected, and group 2 referred to compromised or regional resections. For example, group 2 disease would include grossly resected tumor with microscopic residual disease, completely resected regional disease in which adjacent lymph nodes were involved with tumor, or extension of tumor into adjacent organs. Group 3 disease referred to patients with incomplete resection of the tumor or biopsy only where there was gross residual disease left behind. Finally, group 4 disease included patients with distant metastases at the time of diagnosis (Halperin et al. 1989).

The IRS grouping system proved to be helpful but had many shortcomings. It did not account for the influence of tumor primary location on outcome, the size of the primary tumor, or emphasize the question of nodal involvement. Recently, the IRS has adopted a tumor/node/metastases (TNM) pretreatment staging classification based upon thorough clinical examination, laboratory studies, and imaging examination. Any patient with metastatic disease at presentation is considered stage 4. Patients without metastases who have primary tumors in the orbit, other sites in the head and neck exclusive of parameningeal sites, or genitourinary sites other than the bladder and prostate are stage 1 disease, irrespective of whether the lymph nodes are clinically involved by neoplasm. Patients with prostate or bladder primary sites, extremity sites, parameningeal sites, and other sites such as the trunk, retroperitoneum, etc., are considered to have stage 2 disease if the lymph nodes are not clinically involved or if the clinical status of the regional lymph nodes are unknown. Patients are classified as having stage 3 disease if the lymph nodes are involved and/or the primary tumor is greater than 5 cm in diameter. This patient at presentation would have been group 3 and, presumably, stage 3.

The probability of survival following therapy of RMS is dependent upon tumor site, histologic subtype, and stage/group. Because there is the previously mentioned association between histologic subtype and primary tumor location, as well as an association between primary tumor location and stage/group (i.e., most orbital tumors are in group 3), we may infer that multivariate analysis would be necessary to determine if site, histology, group, or any other factors are independent predictors of outcome. A univariate and multivariate analysis has been conducted of 1688 patients entered on the clinical IRS-1 and IRS-2 studies from 1972 through 1984 (Crist et al. 1990). The median follow-up time for surviving patients is 9 years for IRS-1 and 5 years for IRS-2. Five-year survival for IRS-1 by group is: I, 83%; II, 71%; III, 52%; IV, 21%. Slight improvements were seen in 5-year survivals in IRS-2 for group 3 patients. Survivals were: I, 81%; II, 80%; III, 65%; and IV, 27%. For group 3 head and neck primary RMS above the clavicles, such as in our patient, the IRS-2 five-year survivals were: orbit, 90%, parameningeal sites, 66%, and other head and neck sites, 76%. Similar results have been reported by the Children's Hospital of Philadelphia (Anderson et al. 1990). In a univariant analysis of group 3 RMS such as case 49, alveolar RMS in the IRS did less well than embryonal cases (5-year survival 70% versus 56%) and 5-year survival increased as tumor size decreased (less than 3 cm primary, 83%; 3–5 cm, 73%; greater than 5 cm, 55%; $p < 0.001$) (Crist et al. 1990). In the future "biologic" staging of RMS utilizing DNA ploidy and oncogene amplification may prove to be of additional value in predicting prognosis (Anonymous 1989).

This patient had bilateral nodal involvement at presentation. The incidence of lymph node involvement in RMS is a matter of interest. Although the conventional wisdom is that sarcomas rarely spread to lymphatics, this is often incorrect in RMS (Grieman 1988). In 1977 Lawrence et al. reported a prevalence of lymph node metastases of 19% in genitourinary RMS, 17% in extremity lesions, 10% in trunk primaries, 0% in orbital tumors, and 3% at other head and neck sites (Anderson et al. 1990). Donaldson et al. (1973) reported a 26% (five out of 19) incidence of clinically apparent nodal disease in head and neck primary cases. Jereb et al. (1985) reported a 21% incidence (five out of 23) in non-orbital head and neck tumors. In a series confined to parameningeal RMS, Gasparini et al. (1990) found palpable cervical lymph node metastases in six out of 15 (40%) of cases. Some of the differences in reports concerning the frequency of nodal involvement may be explicable on the basis of the skill and vigor of the examining physician, the frequency of surgical exploration and biopsy of suspicious nodes, as well as the small number of patients in each individual series. In general, in the absence of palpable nodes, neck dissection is not indicated. For palpable nodes, chemotherapy and radiotherapy are utilized to control disease (Anderson et al. 1990).

The debate in recent years concerning the prevention of meningeal dissemination of parameningeal RMS has been instructive and productive. In 1978 TEFFT et al. described 57 patients with parameningeal RMS enrolled in IRS-1. Forty patients were in group 3 and 17 in group 4. Ten patients had meningeal involvement at diagnosis as evidenced by cranial nerve involvement, increase in intracranial pressure, spinal cord compression, and/or positive CSF cytology. Ten other patients developed meningeal involvement during therapy for a total of 20/57 (35%) of parameningeal RMS developing meningeal involvement. Review of the radiotherapy delivered to those children who developed meningeal involvement showed that, in most patients, the irradiated volume was too small or the dose of irradiation was insufficient (less than 50 Gy). The question was raised of whether or not routine prophylactic craniospinal irradiation and intrathecal drugs or cranial irradiation and intrathecal drugs should be considered part of the management of parameningeal RMS (ANONYMOUS 1989). Shortly after the report of TEFFT et al. (1978), CHAN et al. (1979) reported a series of patients with group 3 parameningeal RMS from the MD Anderson Hospital. Only 2.27 (7%) of such patients suffered meningeal relapse. BERRY and JENKIN (1981), of the Princess Margaret Hospital, noted that if one studied the patterns of failure of patients with parameningeal RMS, very few central nervous system (CNS) failures would have been prevented by intrathecal chemotherapy and prophylactic cranial irradiation. Several meningeal failures were the result of relapse at the primary tumor site. In 1985 JEREB et al. reported the Memorial Sloan-Kettering Cancer Center series showing that all patients with parameningeal RMS who suffered CNS relapses also had failure of local control. Whole brain irradiation and/or intrathecal chemotherapy would have been unlikely to influence this occurrence. ANDERSON et al. (1990) found tumor cells in the CSF of one out of 60 patients with head and neck RMS at presentation (2%) and six of ten patients at some point in their illness (10%).

In IRS-2 47 children with parameningeal RMS were prospectively treated with local irradiation, systemic chemotherapy, and a CNS prophylaxis program consisting of craniospinal irradiation and intrathecal methotrexate and hydrocortisone. Only 20 of the 47 patients, however, received spinal axis irradiation and only 12 of those 20 patients received it in accordance with protocol guidelines. The majority of patients were group 3 and there was a 51% 3 year tumor-free survival rate (GASPARINI et al. 1990; RANEY et al. 1992). The increase in survival of patients with parameningeal RMS seen from IRS-1 to IRS-2 may have been partially attributable to the practice of CNS prophylaxis. By the time IRS-III was conducted, however, the widespread availability of tumor imaging with computed tomography (CT) as well as concerns about the toxicity of cranial irradiation prompted a revised strategy.

The IRS-III was designed to limit the volume of tissue irradiated to only the tumor plus margin of adjacent meninges, in those patients with base of skull erosion and/or cranial nerve palsy but without gross cranial extension. Investigators wished to eliminate whole brain radiotherapy for some patients but not jeopardize disease control and survival. Intrathecal chemotherapy was administered to all patients. One hundred and forty-eight patients with parameningeal RMS were entered on the study. The vast majority were group 3. There was an 82% complete response rate and a 9% partial response rate in patients in groups 1, 2, and 3, and a 61% combined complete and partial response rate in group 4. There is an 82% three-year survival rate in groups 1–3, apparently superior to that achieved in IRS-2. Such data might suggest that decreasing the volume of tissue irradiated in patients with parameningeal RMS without intracranial extension does *not* jeopardize disease control or survival (ORTEGA et al. 1990).

GASPARINI et al. (1990) confirmed the findings of IRS-III. They treated 15 cases of parameningeal RMS with intracranial tumor extension, base of skull erosion, and/or cranial nerve palsies. All received systemic or intrathecal chemotherapy along with the irradiation of the local tumor volume with a 2 cm margin. Meningeal involvement and/or progression within the CNS never occurred as a first sign of relapse. Two patients relapsed in the CNS following a local failure. Neither initial prophylactic cranial irradiation nor craniospinal irradiation would have influenced the outcome (GASPARINI et al. 1990).

Contemporary radiotherapy recommendations for primary therapeutic management of parameningeal RMS are that patients with negative CSF cytology, no intracranial extension, no base of skull involvement, and no cranial nerve involvement, or those with no obvious intracranial extension but with limited erosion of the base of skull and/or cranial nerve palsy, ought to receive radiotherapy to the primary tumor site with a 2 cm margin along the base of skull and meninges and around the limits of involvement. Patients with intracranial meningeal extension of tumor in continuity with the primary tumor, with negative CSF cytology, receive irradiation to the primary tumor site plus the intracranial tumor extension with a 2 cm margin. Whole brain irradiation is not administered. This rare patient with diffuse intracranial meningeal extension in continuity with the primary, or multiple sites of brain parenchymal disease, receives whole brain irradiation prior to cone down field directed at the primary tumor. All patients with RMS, of whatever group or site, receive chemotherapy as a crucial component of their overall management.

This patient developed, at 9 months post diagnosis, malignant spinal cord compression at T7 and a positive CSF cytology. Once the tumor relapse was diagnosed, it would have been worthwhile doing a systemic evaluation of the patient to identify other sites of contemporaneous relapse. While the identification of multiple sites of relapse will not materially affect the patient's already dismal prognosis, it would be worthwhile to know what other clinical problems are likely to arise in the coming months.

There are several strong arguments against the use of a posterior laminectomy and decompressive surgery to manage the spinal cord compression. The spinal cord compression exists in the setting of a positive CSF cytology. Thus, a laminectomy will not address the issue of neuraxis dissemination of the tumor. The cure rate of relapsed RMS is, in general, less than 3% (Pizzo et al. 1989). The disease-free survival rate almost exactly corresponds to the overall survival rate (Crist et al. 1990). In view of the very small chance of cure and the very limited life expectancy, expenditure of a large amount of time recuperating from major surgery is not wise. Finally, RMS is a relatively radioresponsive tumor. A palliative response of the spinal cord compression at T7 is just as likely to be obtained by steroids and local irradiation as by decompressive laminectomy, steroids, and postoperative irradiation.

In the radiotherapeutic management of the spinal cord compression at T7, one must consider whether a local irradiation field would be utilized as compared to comprehensive neuroaxis irradiation in view of the positive CSF cytology. Since the patient is extremely unlikely to be cured, and since the acute toxicity of neuroaxis irradiation, following systemic chemotherapy, would be high, I would opt for a local limited field of irradiation to address the acute symptom. I would deal with subsequent metastases in the CNS if and when they arise.

The specifics of the initial chemotherapy administered in this patient are not mentioned. The most commonly used program, however, is vincristine, actinomycin, cyclophosphamide (VAC).s Other agents active in the management of RMS include melphalan, ifosfamide, and etoposide (VP16) either given alone or in combination (Halperin et al. 1989). If one were to adopt an aggressive posture in the management of this patient's relapse, in spite of the data suggesting that the chance of cure is almost zero, then one might propose "salvage" chemotherapy – perhaps in conjunction with granulocyte-colony-stimulating factor to deal with the potential problem of a diminished ability to administer chemotherapy because of prior marrow injury from antecedent chemotherapy. An even more aggressive approach, currently under investigation, is to use high-dose aggressive salvage chemotherapy, sometimes including total body irradiation, with autologous bone marrow rescue. The role of this technique of autologous bone marrow transplantation (ABMT) in RMS is under study. Tumor responses to high-dose cytoreductive therapy have been obtained. The duration of responses have been short. There are, as yet, no long-term disease-free survivors of ABMT for relapsed RMS (Pick 1988; Yaniv et al. 1990).

Whether this case is strictly palliative, as currently available data would suggest, or whether to adopt a more aggressive treatment posture, as hope and prayer may prompt, is dependent upon the expressed wishes of the patient and her family. Due consideration should also be given to whether aggressive "curative" salvage therapy would be given as a component of a clinical study. There is, perhaps, nothing as painful in oncology as the death of a child. It defies rational explanation and calls into question, on the part of the patient, family, and health care providers, a fundamental belief system in a rational and just universe. The treating radiation oncologist must provide compassionate care and guidance and must, to the extent possible, prevent emotion from overcoming sound clinical judgement.

References

Anderson GJ, Tom LWC, Womer RB, Handler SD, Wetmore RF, Potsic WP (1990) Rhabdomyosarcoma of children. Arch Otolaryngol Head Neck Surg 116: 428–431

Anonymous (1989) Prognostic factors in childhood rhabdomyosarcoma. Lancet 2: 959–960

Berry MP, Jenkin RDT (1981) Parameningeal rhabdomyosarcoma in the young. Cancer 48: 281–288

Bonilla JA, Healy GB (1989) Management of malignant head and neck tumors in children. Pediatr Clinic North Am 36: 1443–1450

Chan RC, Sutow WW, Linberg RD (1979) Parameningeal rhabdomyosarcoma. Radiology 131: 211

Crist WM, Gamsey L, Beltangady MS, Mauer HM (1990) Prognosis in children with rhabdomyosarcoma: a report of the intergroup rhabdomyosarcoma studies I and II. J Clin Oncol 8: 443–452

Donaldson S, Castro J, Wilbur J, Jesse R (1973) Rhabdomyosarcoma of head and neck in children. Cancer 31: 26–35

Gasparini M, Lombardi F, Massimino M, Gandola L, Fossati-Bellani F (1990) Questionable role of CNS radioprophylaxis in the therapeutic management of childhood rhabdomyosarcoma with meningeal extension. J Clin Oncol 8: 1854–1857

Grieman RB, Katsikeris NF, Symington JM (1988) Rhabdomyosarcoma of the maxillary sinus: review of the literature and report of a case. J Oral Maxillofac Surg 46: 1090–1096

Halperin EC, Kun LE, Constine LS, Tarbell NJ (1989) Pediatric radiation oncology. Raven, New York, pp 223–246

Jereb B, Haik BG, Ong R, Ghavimi F (1985) Parameningeal rhabdomyosarcoma (including the orbit): results of orbital irradiation. Int J Radiat Oncol Biol Phys 11: 2057–2065

Lawrence W, Hays DM, Moon TE (1977) Lymphatic metastases with childhood rhabdomyosarcoma. Cancer 39: 556–559

MacArthur CJ, McGill TJI, Healy GB (1992) Pediatric head and neck rhabdomyosarcoma. Clin Pediatr 31(2): 66–70

Ortega JA, Fryer E, Gehan P, Jones-Norris P, Raney B, Webber B, Wiener E, Maurer H (1990) Efficacy of reducing tissue volume irradiation in children with cranial (CR) parameningeal (PM) rhabdomyosarcoma (RMS): a report for the intergroup rhabdomyosarcoma study (IRS) III. Proc ASCO, 9: 296

Pick TE (1988) Autologous bone marrow transplantation in children. Crit Rev Oncol Hematol 8: 311–337

Pizzo PA, Horowitz ME, Poplack DG, Hay DM, Kun LE (1989) Solid tumor of childhood. In: DeVita Jr VT, Hellman S, Rosenbery SA (eds) Cancer: principles and practice of oncology. Lippincott, Philadelphia, pp 1612–1670

Raney B, Tefft M, Heyn R, Newton W, Morris Jones P, Haeberlen V, Maurer J (1992) Ascending myelitis after intensive chemotherapy and radiation therapy in children with cranial parameningeal sarcoma. Cancer 69: 1498–1506

Rapidis AD, Economidis J, Goumas PD, Langdon JD, Skordalakis A, Tzortzatou F, Anagnostopoulos D, Mastaniotis N (1988) Tumors of the head and neck in children. J Craniomaxillofac Surg 16: 279–286

Salloum E, Flamant F, Rey A, Caillaud JM, Friedman S, Valteau D, Lemerle J (1989) Rhabdomyosarcoma in infants under one year of age: experience of the Institut Gustave-Roussy. Med Pediatr Oncol 17: 424–428

Schwaab G, Bouzouitak, Janot F, Flamant F, Luboinski B (1989) Les cancers orals de l'enfant. Repartition histologique et topographiqe. Indications therapeutiques. Bull Cancer 76: 757–762

Tefft M, Fernandez C, Donaldson M, Newton W, Moon T (1978) Incidence of meningeal involvement by rhabdomyosarcoma of the head and neck in children. Cancer 42: 254–258

Yaniv I, Bouffet E, Irle C, Negrier S, Biron P, Favrot M, Phillip I, Brunat-Mentigny M, Phillip T (1990) Autologous bone marrow transplantation in pediatric solid tumors. Pediatr Hematol Oncol 7: 35–46

2 Advanced Cancer of the Hypopharynx

L.J. PETERS and H. GOEPFERT

A 65-year-old man presented with T3N3 squamous cell carcinoma of the pyriform sinus. He was given 70 Gy in 35 fractions with incomplete resolution of the primary and nodal masses. Since irradiation, the patient has been able to eat soft foods with difficulty and has lost weight. One month after irradiation, a Hickman catheter was placed for total parenteral nutrition (TPN), and chemotherapy was given. Chemotherapy had to be discontinued because of pneumonia associated with severe neutropenia. Chemotherapy could not be restarted, the lesions began to grow again, and he left the hospital after 3 weeks on TPN and morphine.

1. Should all *advanced* pyriform sinus tumors be treated? What if there were no evidence of metastases?
2. Does chemotherapy benefit patients with radioresistant tumors?
3. When should TPN be used?

Response

The above vignette illustrates a situation too often encountered in oncology where sequential treatments with little or no likelihood of benefitting a patient are offered merely because the modalities exist. In academic institutions, there may be further steps in the process where patients who have progressive disease after conventional treatment are enrolled on Phase I/II research protocols to evaluate their response to investigational agents. Having a large number of therapeutic options allows physicians to tell patients confidently that there is always "something more that can be done." While this may be reassuring to the patient's relatives, and even transiently to the patient, it is doubtful whether continued therapeutic intervention is preferable to symptomatic terminal care in the majority of cases of this type. The vignette described raises several important medical and ethical questions.

Was The Initial Treatment Intent Clearly Defined?

We are presented with a 65-year-old man with an advanced carcinoma of the pyriform sinus with extensive neck disease. We are not told of his general condition prior to radiotherapy, but can surmise that he would have lost weight and be in a somewhat debilitated condition. In such a patient, the probability of securing local-regional control with radiotherapy alone is slim (BATAINI et al. 1982), and one must question the wisdom of the decision to offer radical radiotherapy as definitive treatment. Since the best (albeit still suboptimal) chance of securing local regional control in such a patient is with surgical resection followed by postoperative radiotherapy, one wonders why this strategy was not followed. Quite possibly, the patient was deemed "inoperable" by a consulting surgeon. Inoperability is, however, a vague term, often used incorrectly as a synonym for unresectability, and very subjectively applied. In our view, a patient should not be assessed as unresectable until he has been evaluated by an experienced oncologic head and neck surgeon. An expert surgical opinion is crucial in assessing the potential benefits of large operations. While resection of advanced tumors (usually with postoperative radiotherapy) is often the best way to alleviate the symptoms of such tumors, this is true only if local regional control is secured. Clearly, there is no benefit to the patient from heroic operations which do not achieve this goal. The best surgeon is one who combines technical virtuosity with an ability to recognize his/her limitations and who does not allow professional ego to affect his/her decision making.

Whether the patient in our vignette was medically fit for surgery is another question. It is interesting

Lester J. Peters, MD, Professor and Director, Division of Radiotherapy, The University of Texas, MD Anderson Cancer Center, Box 97, 1515 Holcombe Boulevard, Houston, TX 77030–4095, USA

Helmuth Goepfert, MD, Professor and Chairman, Department of Head and Neck Surgery, The University of Texas, MD Anderson Cancer Center, 1515 Holcombe Boulevard, Houston, TX 77030–4095, USA

that after unsuccessful radiotherapy, the patient was given TPN. If surgery was contraindicated initially on the basis of his general condition, it would have been far preferable to have used TPN than to improve the patient's physiological status to enable surgery to be performed if curative treatment was seriously considered. We cannot emphasize too strongly the point that the only real prospect of controlling advanced head and neck cancer is with the initial therapeutic intervention, often with combined modalities. Salvage after failed initial treatment is rarely, if ever, achieved.

How Does One Decide If Attempted Cure Is Reasonable?

This is a difficult philosophical decision which must be based on more than mere assessment of tumor extent, although the latter is an essential prerequisite. To enable a rational decision to be made, it is important that a detailed evaluation of the extent of local and regional disease be undertaken along with a chest X-ray to rule-out preexisting metastatic disease and/or primary lung cancer. Even with a negative chest X-ray, it is quite likely that a patient with a primary hypopharyngeal cancer and advanced neck disease will, in truth, have micrometastatic disease. However, this becomes an issue in terms of survival only if the local and regional disease is controlled. Further, achieving local and regional control is the best form of symptomatic relief, and will usually provide a better quality of death for incurable patients (from metastatic disease rather than uncontrolled primary disease). Surgical resection will, however, necessitate a laryngectomy, and the patient's literacy and social support system are important factors to consider in terms of rehabilitation.

To summarize, it is vitally important that a clear and conscious choice be made between attempted cure or symptomatic treatment only, before embarking on a course of action. If the choice is for attempted cure, then the best and most aggressive treatment should be delivered. It is too easy, as our vignette illustrates, to offer treatment with little or no chance of success and continue, with ever-decreasing return, to dig a deeper oncologic hole.

Options for Curative Treatment

Data from MD Anderson indicate that patients of this type treated by surgical resection and postoperative radiotherapy have a 2-year probability of local and regional disease control of approximately 70% (PETERS et al. 1993). This contrasts with a chance of perhaps 20% with radiotherapy alone. The use of induction chemotherapy prior to definitive treatment has been shown in many clinical trials not to improve overall local control rates or survival (STELL and RAWSON 1990). However, this treatment strategy can be used as a selection process to identify patients in whom laryngectomy might be avoided (WOLF et al. 1991). It is reasonable, therefore, especially in patients who are poorly equipped to cope with a laryngectomy, to use induction chemotherapy with the understanding that surgery must still follow unless there is a complete, or near complete response.

Digging the Oncologic Hole

In the vignette, we are told that after a poor response to radiotherapy, the patient was offered chemotherapy along with TPN 1 month later. There are absolutely no data to justify the use of chemotherapy under such circumstances. The likelihood of achieving a complete response after unsuccessful radical radiotherapy is very small, and whatever transient responses are achieved are of short duration (WOLF et al. 1991). Administering chemotherapy under such circumstances might be termed cruel and unusual punishment, and is therefore banned by the United States Constitution! As previously stated, it is not justified to offer treatment merely on the grounds that it has not previously been used. In our view, the patient with massive residual disease after radiotherapy is unsalvageable, and should be offered supportive care only. Whether this includes TPN or a feeding gastrostomy is highly debatable. Often, these measures simply prolong life while adding nothing to its quality. We would submit that there are very few circumstances where TPN can be justified in a patient with inevitably fatal disease in whom local disease progression adds nothing but misery to what life remains. Equally unjustified in our view is intensive antibiotic therapy for pneumonia, and, of course, resuscitation following cardiopulmonary arrest. Insidiously, each step taken to prolong life makes withholding the next step more difficult. A commitment once made is hard to revoke.

The issue of prolonging life is similar in many ways to that of initial treatment. It is easy to embark on a course of action, but far more difficult to extricate oneself from an ill-chosen course. How easy it is to wash one's hands of a painful decision of this type by simply telling the patient that he is eligible for a trial of a new drug/biological. Because a patient's death signifies treatment "failure," we understandably feel professionally inadequate and resentful about the outcome, and seek to avoid defeat by launching another offensive against the cancer. But is it in the patient's best interest? A sound criterion is to ask two questions of oneself: (a) would I accept this treatment myself if I were in the patient's situation? and (b) am I making this treatment recommendation because I fully believe it will help the patient or because I do not want to admit to therapeutic impotence? Too often, we jump into action for the latter reason, and because we lack the training and experience to deal with the medical and emotional needs of dying patients and their families. To quote Thomas Mann, "Death is more dreadful for the surviving than for the dying."

In our view, most patients would far prefer to be given a compassionate but realistic assessment of the way in which their disease is likely to progress, reassurance that control of pain is almost always possible, and comfort that they will not be abandoned in the dying process. The popularity of Living Wills and similar instruments is testimony to the fact that many patients wish to be spared heroic efforts to prolong life when their outlook is hopeless. We as physicians must respect their wishes.

Control of Pain

There is a curious reluctance in the medical community to prescribe sufficient doses of narcotics for patients with incurable cancer (WANGER et al. 1989). This phenomenon has been described many times, but nonetheless persists, probably because of the image of narcotic use portrayed by the Drug Enforcement Administration. It is unconscionable to prescribe doses of narcotics insufficient to achieve pain relief on the grounds that a patient with incurable cancer may become addicted. Whenever a patient is discharged to another physician for terminal care, it is essential that advice be given by the oncologist regarding appropriate doses and schedule of pain medication. This is truly the last and greatest service we can give to patients who cannot be cured.

Economic Considerations

With the cost of health care completely out of control, and now consuming 13% of the country's Gross National Product, it is imperative that medical resources be allocated to where they will be best spent. Hospitalizing a patient such as the one described in our vignette for TPN and chemotherapy is an example of wasted resources since the cost-benefit ratio is close to infinite (the benefit being essentially nil). As a society, we need to realize that the cost of futile medical intervention is ultimately borne by everyone in the form of higher insurance premiums, increased taxes to support government-sponsored health care programs, and/or reduction in services to the needy if budgetary caps are applied. Further, excessive government spending on medicine means that fewer tax dollars are available for other societal priorities.

At the personal level, families are all too often financially devastated by the cost of expensive therapeutic interventions in incurable situations. In our experience, families are rarely, if ever, told of the financial implications of proceeding with treatment and, indeed, are often passively made to feel guilty if they suggest withholding last-ditch treatment attempts.

Conclusions

This case illustrates, in our view, improper oncologic management in the following aspects.

1. Lack of clear definition of the objectives of treatment before it was embarked upon.
2. The administration of chemotherapy following unsuccessful radiotherapy with essentially no chance of producing a durable remission.
3. The use of TPN as a support system in a patient with incurable disease.

We submit that the patient in this vignette would have been better served by a more aggressive initial treatment approach, and a less aggressive (and less prolonged) approach to postdefinitive therapy. The best oncologist is one who under-stands his abilities and limitations. To acknowledge limitations is not to be nihilistic. Far from it. Modern oncologic practice is heavily oriented towards maximizing treatment with the objective of improving cure rates, and we can claim success in many diseases with this approach. A corollary, however, which is much less widely accepted, is that there is a time to concede defeat before a patient is treated into the grave. More emphasis needs to be placed on training oncologists to deal with the medical and emotional needs of dying patients and their families.

References

Bataini P, Brugere J, Bernier J, Jaulerry CH, Picot C, Ghossein NA (1982) Results of radical radiotherapeutic treatment of carcinoma of the pyriform sinus. Experience of the Institut Curie. Int J Radiat Oncol Biol Phys 8: 1277–1286

Peters LJ, Goepfert H, Ang KK, Byers RM, Maor MH, Guillamondegui O, Morrison WH, Weber RS, Garden AS, Frankenthaler RA, Oswald MJ, Brown BW (1993) Evaluation of the dose for postoperative radiation therapy of head and neck cancer. First report of a prospective randomized trial. Int J Radiat Oncol Biol Phys 26: 3–11

Stell PM, Rawson NSB (1990) Adjuvant chemotherapy in head and neck cancer. Br J Cancer 61: 779–787

Wanger SH, Federman DD, Adelstein SJ et al. (1989) The physician's responsibility towards hopelessly ill patients. N Engl J Med 320: 844–940

Wolf G, Lippman SM, Laramore G, Hong WK (1991) Head and neck cancer. In: Holland JF, Frei E, Bast RC Jr, Kufe DW, Morton DL, Weichselbaum R (eds) Cancer medicine, 3rd edn. Lea and Febiger, Philadelphia

Wolf GT et al. (members of the Department of Veteran's Affairs, Laryngeal Cancer Study Group) (1991) Induction chemotherapy plus radiation compared with surgery plus radiation in patients with advanced laryngeal cancer. N Engl J Med 324: 1685–1690

3 Paraplegia

J.F. Wilson and K. Murray

The patient was a 40-year-old woman who had been complaining of progressive lumbar back pain for 2 years. Finally, after paraplegia, a lumbar paraspinous mass was noted, fine-needle aspirate showed lymphocytes associated with other inflammatory cells. Due to a change in mental state, a computed tomography (CT) scan of the brain was taken, and this showed multiple large solid and cavitary lesions. The patient responded poorly to dexamethasone (Decadron). Repeat biopsy of the paraspinal mass showed large cell lymphoma.

She was in semicoma and disoriented, and her gag reflex was intact. Her axillary femoral bypass graft was functioning.

1. Would you irradiate this patient's brain or paraspinal mass?
2. What is your experience with patients whose neurologic symptoms do not respond to steroids?
3. If you could not stabilize her head movement, would that change your plan to irradiate?
4. [Include other considerations that would influence your recommendation]

Response

To summarize, this patient has a large paraspinal mass, progressive back pain, paraplegia, change in mental status, and multiple intracranial lesions. A biopsy of the paraspinal mass has demonstrated a large cell lymphoma and it is assumed her intracranial disease is a manifestation of the same neoplasm. To date, her only therapeutic intervention has been a trial of Decadron and she is noted to have responded poorly to this. We would definitely recommend radiation therapy for this patient, both to the paraspinous mass as well as to the intracranial lesions. The main goal of this therapy would be to reverse her two neurologic problems of paraplegia and acute mental status change. The potential advantages of successful treatment of such a patient are self-evident although the overall prognosis may remain poor. In the absence of information relative to the patient's general status or knowledge of any advance directives given by the patient, we would proceed. Decompressive surgery such as a laminectomy could also be considered especially if there is radiographic evidence of bony fragments causing impingement on the spinal cord. However, Young et al. (1980), in a randomized trial comparing laminectomy and postoperative irradiation with external beam radiation alone, found no significant difference in the two treatment methods in regards to pain relief, improved ambulation, or improved sphincter function. Additionally, proceeding with external beam irradiation initially to try to provide a maximal reduction in the size of this disease (which is generally relatively radiosensitive). Previous experience with extradural lymphomas has indicated a maintenance or return to normal ambulatory function in 90% (19 of 21) of cases treated (Rathmell et al. 1992). Systemic management with chemotherapy remains an important therapeutic option in patients with advanced malignant lymphomas and will also need to be considered in this particular patient.

The patient's past history of vascular surgery is certainly interesting. A possibility of previous blood transfusions in the past must be considered, as it potentially raises the question of human immunodeficiency virus (HIV) status. Rapid dissemination of malignant lymphoma can be seen in patients who are HIV-positive. Therefore, we would also recommend testing this patient for HIV. This would also have some bearing on this patient's treatment plan. Patients treated for Kaposi's sarcoma who have a past history of infection from HIV and receive treatment to the oral cavity can develop an intolerable mucositis after only a few gray (Cooper

J. Frank Wilson, MD, FACR, Professor and Chairman, Dept Radiation Oncology, Milwaukee County Medical Complex, Milwaukee, WI 53226, USA
Kevin Murray, MD, Assistant Professor, Radiation Oncology, Medical College of Wisconsin, 8700 West Wisconsin Avenue, Milwaukee, WI 53226, USA

et al. 1988; Watkins et al. 1987). While this has been demonstrated mainly in oropharyngeal mucosa, effects on the gastrointestinal (GI) tract may also need to be examined.

We would recommend treating the whole brain using opposed lateral treatment fields and separate treatment fields for the paraspinous mass. Craniospinal irradiation could be considered since the most likely route of tumor dissemination has been through the cerebrospinal fluid (CSF). However, her confusion would make the technical setup for craniospinal irradiation difficult, if not impossible. Additionally, because systemic management with chemotherapy may also be initiated, we would minimize the amount of bone marrow treated by confining our treatment to the cranium and paraspinous mass.

Generally, we would utilize clinically oriented right and left lateral treatment fields. The main limitations of this approach would be the possible underdosing of the anterior aspect of the middle cranial fossa. If this is demonstrated by treatment verification films, we would recommend simulating the patient so that custom blocks can be used to include this meningeal area. Her paraspinous mass would be treated either with a single posteroanterior (PA) treatment field or, if the mass extends sufficiently anteriorly, anteroposterior/posteroanterior (AP/PA) field arrangements could be utilized. With a goal of her therapy to maximize the improvement in her neurologic function within a minimum time period, relatively large fraction sizes of 250–300 cGy per day would be utilized to the cranial fields. This dose would be defined at midline. After a total dose of 30–35 Gy, if there has been a substantial improvement in her neurologic function, reduced treatment fields could then be utilized to boost the actual involved areas to approximately 45 Gy. A fraction size of 300 cGy would be utilized for her paraspinous mass if a single PA treatment field was utilized. If AP/PA treatment fields were required, a slightly lower fraction size of 250 cGy would be utilized to try to minimize acute GI toxicity. A total dose of 25–35 Gy would be given dependent on neurologic improvement.

Ideally, the patient would be treated in the supine position on the treatment table. Stabilization of the head and body could be done with seat belts, masking tape and a nose piece. However, if her level of cooperation is more uncertain, more restrictive devices such as an alpha cradle or aquaplast could be utilized. Additionally, a mild degree of sedation could be provided through the use of midazolam (Versed). If the patient's level of confusion and disorientation could not be sufficiently controlled with low-dose Versed, a deeper level of sedation could be provided with the support of the department of anesthesia. If the patient's general medical status is not a candidate for anesthesia support, the ability to provide external beam irradiation in a precise and reproducible manner would be compromised and we would then suggest proceeding with systemic chemotherapy.

As her external beam irradiation is proceeding, if the patient is showing significant neurologic improvement, a workup for the extent of her disease needs to be completed. This would include a bilateral bone marrow aspirate and biopsies, routine laboratory studies including a complete blood count, liver function studies (especially lactate dehydrogenase), a chest X-ray, and a CT scan of the chest, abdomen and pelvis.

References

Cooper JS, Fried PR (1988) Case report. Treatment of aggressive epidemic Kaposi's sarcoma of the conjunctiva by radiotherapy. Arch Ophthalmol 106(1): 20–21

Rathmell AJ, Gospodarowicz MK, Sutcliffe SB, Clark RM, et al. (1992) Localized extradural lymphoma: survival, relapse pattern and functional outcome. The Princess Margaret Hospital Lymphoma Group. Radiother Oncol 24(1): 14–20

Watkins EB, Findley P, Gelmann E, et al. (1987) Enhanced mucosal reactions in AIDS patients receiving oropharyngeal irradiation. Comment. Int J Radiat Oncol Biol Phys 13(9): 1403–1408

Young RF, Post EM, King GA (1980) Treatment of spinal epidural metastases. Randomized prospective comparison of laminectomy and radiotherapy. J Neurosurg 53(6): 741–748

4 Melanomatosis with Abnormal Cerebral Computed Tomography Scan

M. RYOO

A 78-year-old man had a routine chest radiograph which showed two nodules in the left lower lung. Computed tomography (CT) demonstrated one of the nodules to be subpleural. Over the ensuing 2 months, these nodules grew; CT-guided needle biopsy was not diagnostic. Four months after the CT-guided needle biopsy, a left posterolateral thoracotomy revealed three separate lung lesions. Histopathology was malignant melanoma. Postoperatively, a cerebral CT scan in this asymptomatic patient showed a left frontal and a right posterior occipital lesion compatible with metastases.

1. What treatment would you recommend?
2. What is to be gained by actively treating this patient now?
3. Would a positive CT brain scan earlier have precluded the thoracotomy?
4. [Include other considerations that would influence your recommendation].

Response

I would not recommend any active treatment to this man because he is asymptomatic in spite of melanomatosis to the lung and brain. When one is faced with an incurable patient, the goal of management is palliative; the treatment should be rendered to relieve particular symptoms in order to improve the quality of life rather than to prolong life with iatrogenic illnesses. The medial survival for disseminated melanoma is often short. Most of the literature reports less than 6 months of survival time in patients with melanoma in the central nervous system (CNS) (CHOI et al. 1985; STRIDSKLEV et al. 1984; MENDEZ and DELMAESTRO 1988; RATE et al. 1988). There are no prognostic factors which are agreed upon by all studies but if the disease-free interval from the primary to the metastasis is long, the metastasis is solitary and only one metastatic deposit is present, my strategy, depending upon the general condition of the patient might be different. Sometimes other primaries such as metastatic kidney or thyroid cancer may have a slower pace. However, multiple metastatic foci of melanoma in the CNS are fatal, relatively quickly. The cause of death in most patients is progressive intracranial melanoma. There have been clinical reports of retrospective studies evaluating the role of craniotomy (NEUSS et al. 1990; OREDESSON et al. 1990; WORNOM et al. 1986), radiation treatment with or without craniotomy (CHOI et al. 1985; STRIDSKLEV et al. 1984; MENDEZ and DELMAESTRO 1988; RATE et al. 1988), and chemo-therapy (JACQUILLAT et al. 1990). My review of the literature leads me to conclude that "gained" survival in one subset of patients over the other is due to patient selection rather that the superiority of one treatment over another. Accordingly, I would also conclude that there is no widely accepted single treatment regimen in CNS melanoma.

There is no active gain by treating this patient now, in my opinion. The only rationalization one might imagine in treating him now is based on a hope (or an anecdotal, personal case) that treatment may prolong the asymptomatic period for an indeterminate length of time. Are there scientific data supporting this rationale? Not to my knowledge! One might argue that radiation is more effective when utilized early when there is small tumor burden (microscopic disease) in the asymptomatic patient.

We reviewed the outcome in 56 symptomatic patients with CNS melanoma who were treated with large fractions of megavoltage irradiation between 1975 and 1989 at our institution (RYOO et al. 1990). All but eight patients received a tumor dose of 2000 cGy in five equal fractions in 5–8 days. One patient had 3000 cGy in ten fractions, four had 4000 cGy in eight fractions in a split fashion, two had 5120 cGy in 32 fractions, and one died after treatment. Eighteen patients (32%) underwent craniotomy for decompression or diagnosis prior to irradiation.

Monica Ryoo, MD, Radiation Oncology Department, Southern California Permanente Medical Group, 4950 Sunset Boulevard, Los Angeles, CA 90027, USA

Table 1. Comparison of treatment, favorable factors, and survival

Reference	Most common dose			Favorable factors	Median survival (months)
	Total (rad)	Weekly (rad)	Fraction number		
1	3000–4800	300–240	10–20 b.i.d.	Complete resection No extraneural metastasis	3
2	3300	2400	7	33.6 Gy in 7 fractions with chemotherapy[a]	2
3	mean 3000	n/a	n/a	Surgery for solitary lesion without irradiation[b]	3
4	3000	1000–1200	5–6	Single lesion resection[c]	3.5
9	2000	n/a	5	Craniotomy in solitary lesion KS 70%–100%	3

n/a, not available; KS, Karnofsky status
[a] Chemotherapy with lomustine (CCNU), vincristine, dacarbazine (DTIC).
[b] Twice per week treatment.
[c] Patients treated with chemotherapy fared worse.

Forty-seven patients (84%) had extraneural melanoma as well as CNS metastasis. Approximately 30% of 18 patients who underwent craniotomy had Karnofsky Status (KS) of 70%– 100%, 40% had KS of 50%–60%. The patients who underwent irradiation only had a relatively lower KS that of the craniotomy group.

Table 1 summarizes the result relative to radiation dose, median survival and favorable prognostic factors (Choi et al. 1985; Stridsklev et al. 1984; Mendez and DelMaestro 1988; Rate et al. 1988; Ryoo et al. 1990). As shown in this table, overall median survival time is similar regardless of total tumor dose or fractionation.

Would a positive CT brain scan earlier have precluded the thoracotomy? Most probably, yes. There are few curable cancers which are metastatic to lung and brain in a 78-year-old man. Pancreatic and pulmonary cancer have the highest incidence and are incurable. Lymphoma is an important diagnosis to exclude. Knowing the presence of cerebral metastasis would have helped me insist on repeated percutaneous pleural biopsies or thoracoscopy, rather than thoracotomy. Other primaries besides lymphoma to consider for which there is effective systemic management is breast or prostate cancer. Breast cancer in the male is not occult, and prostate cancer metastasize widely to bone (including the epidural spaces). Germ cell tumors are unlikely in this age group but could be excluded by alpha-feta protein and chorio-gonadotrophin titers. In summary, I would consider management for symptoms only in this patient, being careful not to create any iatrogenic illnesses.

References

Choi KN, Withers HR, Rotman M (1985) Intracranial metastases from melanoma: clinical features and treatment by accelerated fractionation. Cancer 56: 1–9
Jacquillat C, Khayat D, Banzet P et al. (1990) Chemotherapy by fotemustine in cerebral metastases of disseminated malignant melanoma. Cancer Chemother Pharmacol 25: 263–266
Mendez IM, DelMaestro RF (1988) Cerebral metastases from malignant melanoma. Can J Neurol Sci 15: 119–123
Neuss M, Konig A, Herrmann H-D (1990) Intracranial melanoma metastases: surgical treatment and follow-up of 18 patients. Anticancer Res 7: 445–446
Oredesson S, Ingvar C, Stromblad L-G, Jonsson P-E (1990) Palliative surgery for brain metastases of malignant melanoma. Eur J Surg Oncol 16: 451–456
Rate WR, Solin LJ, Turrisi AT (1988) Palliative radiotherapy for metastatic malignant melanoma: brain metastases, bone metastases, and spinal cord compression. Int J Radiat Oncol Biol Phys 15: 859–864
Ryoo MC, Kagan AR, Wollin M (1990) Large fraction treatment of 59 patients with metastatic melanoma to the brain (1968–1989). Presented at the Annual RSNA meeting, Chicago, Illinois 1990 (revised)
Stridsklev IC, Hagen S, Klepp O (1984) Radiation therapy for brain metastases from malignant melanoma. Acta Radiol Oncol 23: 231–235
Wornom IL III, Soong S-J, Urist MM, Smith JW, McElvein R, Balch CM (1986) Surgery as palliative treatment for distant metastases of melanoma. Ann Surg 204: 181–185

5 Multiple Cerebral Metastasis from Cancer of the Lung

M. Raben

A 54-year-old white man presented with slurred speech and weakness of his right hand. Magnetic resonance imaging (MRI) showed multiple enhancing lesions in the cerebellum and in the left occipital and left parietal regions. A computerized axial tomography (CAT) scan of the chest showed two nodular lesions in the right lower lobe with a 3 cm ipsilateral mediastinal lymph node. A right transbronchial biopsy revealed poorly differentiated carcinoma. His neurologic symptoms improved on dexamethasone (Decadron).

1. What are your goals in stage IV non-oat cell cancer of the lung with respect to the possible use of radiation and/or chemotherapy?
2. Should patients like this be kept on steroids alone?
3. Would you irradiate the brain now or later?
4. What dose – time regimen do you use?
5. Would you irradiate both lung and brain? Why?
6. [Include other considerations that would influence your recommendations].

Response

In our clinic 20 out of 100 patients seen in consultation for the first time have been referred for us to consider treatment of a metastatic deposit. Sixteen patients will have a documented primary lesion. In four patients the primary will remain unknown. I think the mix and match of patients in our clinic is not too different from that found in other departments. This is the sort of problem all of us face each day.

The probability is that we are dealing with a patient who is not curable. Should we proceed with additional studies to document the extent of his disease? First, of course, I would take a history and examine the patient. In doing this I am looking for the cheapest way to determine other sites of disease and even a primary other than lung cancer, i.e., an enlarged testicle, hemoccult-positive stool, enlarged liver, a suspicious skin lesion, etc. Assuming nothing new is found I would stop at this point and meet with the patient and family.

The purpose of my initial meeting would be to discuss the findings to date, to answer questions which they might have and, most importantly, to establish a relationship with the patient and his family. I would then recommend a course of irradiation (3000 rad in ten fractions) to the brain and the lung even though the latter areas of disease are asymptomatic. I would discuss the physical details the patient would have to go through in the planning and implementation of treatment and acute side effects of therapy. I would then give everyone an opportunity to ask questions.

Usually in my experience while the family will ask questions the patient assumes the position of a disinterested observer. He is not. The probability is that he is in the denial stage of his disease. Interestingly enough, family members may be in other stages of psychological adaptations to this devastating news, for example, the wife is bargaining "we will do anything to get my husband well..." or a son may show anger perhaps because of a feeling of hopelessness that he cannot actively help his father. We not uncommonly find ourselves with a range of emotions all in one room. It is important to deal with each person without leaving the patient out of the picture. It is not uncommon to observe a trainee spend most of the consultative session talking to the family without looking at the patient who continues to maintain this apparent disassociative stance. When the tempo of questions slows down, I suggest that the patient take the day to think about my recommendations. I give them my office number and urge that they call me if further questions come to mind as they invariably do. I arrange for simulation time but explain to the patient that this is merely to expedite the treatment process should he decide to accept my advice. At this point I am talking to the patient, not the family, as

Milton Raben, MD, Department of Radiation Oncology, The Bowman Gray School of Medicine, 300 S. Hawthorne Road, Winston-Salem, NC 27175, USA

I want him to feel that he (as much as possible) is in control of the decision making process. Finally, I offer to help arrange for a second opinion should they want one.

Most patients follow through on the recommended treatment. At the completion of therapy it helps to contact the family physician both by letter and telephone as to the patient's status and what one might expect in the future. A single post-treatment visit will suffice to check for any untoward reactions and then the patient can be seen if necessary at his physician's request.

6 Superior Vena Cava Syndrome

J.E. Marks

Three years ago, a 71-year-old man had a small cell carcinoma of his parotid managed by superficial parotidectomy and postoperative irradiation (6000 cGy at the 80% isodose line with mixed beam). He now presents with a superior vena cava syndrome. Computed tomography (CT) of the chest with IV contrast showed adlenopathy from the level of C3 to the right pulmonary artery, with thrombosis of the right jugular vein. CT-directed needle aspiration of the right peritracheal mass showed small cell carcinoma. He was treated with cyclophosphamide (Cytoxan), doxorubicin (Adriamycin), vincristine and prednisone with a partial response after the first course.

1. Would you irradiate this patient? When? Any adjustment needed because of overlap due to previous irradiation or Adriamycin?
2. Was the chemotherapy indicated? Should it be stopped?
3. [Include other considerations that would influence your recommendation].

Response

The palliative management of patients with advanced malignancy who have received previous irradiation and chemotherapy is a challenging exercise in decision-making. The decisions depend on clinical estimates of life expectancy, tempo of the disease process, and a fundamental knowledge of the potential toxicities of radiation and chemotherapy alone or in combination.

To Irradiate or Not To Irradiate?

A thorough history and physical examination to gain an understanding of previous treatment and current problems is an essential first step in the palliative management of such a case. This patient presents with clinical and radiographic evidence of superior vena caval syndrome and for that reason was referred to radiotherapy. He presumably has discrete signs and symptoms that might be alleviated by irradiating the metastatic lymphadenopathy in the lower neck, thoracic inlet and mediastinum. I would therefore choose to irradiate because radiation will shrink the lymph nodes in the majority of such patients, alleviate their signs and symptoms, and effectively improve their quality of life (Armstrong et al. 1987).

What To Irradiate?

This particular patient has been previously irradiated after superficial parotidectomy for a small carcinoma of the parotid. It is essential in all such cases to obtain the previous radiation records and portal films to determine what was irradiated and how much radiation was given to critical normal structures. In this case, it is essential to determine the inferior margin of the parotid portal and to understand how much radiation was delivered to the spinal cord. Once that is known, it will be possible to shield the spinal cord at the junction of the parotid portal above and the superior vena caval portal below, and thereby avoid radiation myelopathy due to excessive dose at the junction of the two fields. It is often difficult but most important to retrieve the previous records and portal films before planning the radiation treatment. A phone call to the previous radiotherapist is most helpful. Records can be immediately faxed and families are usually more that willing to retrieve the portal films and records. Once the records and films have been obtained, it is an easy matter to shield the spinal cord and construct a portal to include the obstructing lymphadenopathy in the lower neck, thoracic inlet and mediastinum.

James E. Marks, MD, Department of Radiotherapy, Loyola University Medical Center, 2160 S. First Avenue, Maywood, IL 60153, USA

Selection of Dose, Time, and Fractionation

The decision depends on clinical estimates of life expectancy and tempo of disease, the interval from initial presentation to the malignant process or the growth rate of the tumor. This particular patient presented with superior vena cava syndrome some 3 years after his initial surgery and radiation. One might therefore infer that the nature of the disease process is somewhere between indolent and aggressive. Certainly, the patient did not succumb within the year after the initial treatment and may well live another year if effective palliation is achieved. Prescription of dose, time, and fractionation for the palliative management of patients with advanced malignancy ranges from intensive to protracted delivery of dose and depends on clinical estimates of life expectancy. Those with limited life expectancy should be irradiated in an expeditious manner so as not to occupy a great proportion of their remaining life making trips to the radiotherapy department while those who are likely to live a long time can be irradiated in a protracted manner. Conventional fractionization and delivery of a higher dose to eradicate or delay regrowth of tumor for a longer period lessens the likelihood of late effects due to large-fraction irradiation.

Choice of total dose and fractionation also depends on previous or concurrent chemotherapy. Cisplatin and etoposide concurrent with conventional fractionated irradiation 1.8 Gy per day to a total dose of 45–50.5 Gy in 25–28 fractions is well-tolerated and does not generally necessitate interruption of radiation for acute toxicity. Cisplatin and 5-fluorouracil, on the other hand, may cause an acute esophagitis and tracheitis associated with neutropenic fever when used concurrently with fractionated irradiation of the chest. Adriamycin before or during irradiation of the chest is potentially the most dangerous of the combined modality treatments. Anthracyclines cause vacuolization of cardiac myocytes, while radiation alters the fine vasculoconnective stroma of the myocardium (Rubin 1984). Anthracycline cardiomyopathy and radiation cardiomyopathy are both dose-dependent. It is therefore important for the radiotherapist to assess the amount of Adriamycin given and to plan radiation in a less aggressive manner than usual. If the amount of Adriamycin exceeds 400 mg/m^2 and tests of cardiac output show impaired function, one might choose not to irradiate. If the patient has only received 200 mg/m^2 Adriamycin and has normal left ventricular ejection fraction without a history of coronary artery disease, then fractionated irradiation of the mediastinum with shielding of as much heart as possible after 30.6 Gy in 3.5 weeks is probably safe. The final 20 Gy to the upper third of the heart is generally well-tolerated. The combined effects of Adriamycin and radiation on the heart is greater than either modality alone (Eltringham et al. 1975) but an isobologram quantitating the exact amount of drug and radiation that would injure the myocardium in 10% of cases is lacking (Steel 1979).

Summary

I think I would choose protracted delivery of dose in this particular case because of the long interval between initial treatment and recrudescence of disease and the overlapping toxicities of Adriamycin and radiation on the heart (Eltringham et al. 1975). I would prescribe 50 Gy in 5 or 5.5. weeks and carefully shield as much of the heart as possible. My goal would be to keep the patient symptom and sign-free of superior vena caval obstruction for the remainder of his life with the expectation that he might die from inanition that often accompanies disseminated cancer.

References

Armstrong CA, Perez CA, Simpson JR, Hedeman MA (1987) Role of irradiation in the management of superior vena caval syndrome. Int J Radiat Oncol Biol Phys 13: 531–539

Eltringham JR, Fajarado LF, Stewart JR (1975) Adriamycin cardiomyopathy: enhanced cardiac damage in rabbits with combined drug and cardiac irradiation. Radiology 115: 471–472

Rubin P (1984) The Franz Bushke lecture: late effects of chemotherapy and radiation therapy: a new hypothesis. Int J Radiat Oncol Biol Phys 10: 5–34

Steel GG (1979) Terminology in the description of drug-radiation interactions. Int J Radiat Oncol Biol Phys 5: 1145–1150

7 Widely Disseminated Breast Cancer and Hypercalcemia

J. Tsao

Seven years ago, this 48-year-old black woman had a T2N0 adenocarcinoma of the right breast treated by modified radical mastectomy. Four years ago she had a chest wall recurrence which was treated with chemotherapy. For the past 2 weeks she has been bedridden from pain in her hip and bilateral leg weakness. She also has experienced pain in the left shoulder region, lumbar spine, and left anterior lower ribs. Bone scan and X-rays show widespread metastases with an elevated calcium level of 15.6 mg/dl. Chest radiographs show masses in the mediastinum, and computed tomography (CT) of the liver reveals multiple metastases. The hemoglobin level is 9 g/dl and the potassium level 2.9 meq/l.

1. Would you irradiate symptomatic areas only? What dose – time (800 rad in one fraction?)
2. Is magnetic resonance imaging (MRI) of the spinal column indicated?
3. Is hemibody irradiation indicated? How would you plan the junction Welds if there is cord compression at T12–L1?
4. Would a history of previous doxorubicin (Adriamycin) change your recommendations?
5. [Include other considerations that would influence your recommendation].

Response

The decisions regarding palliative management of metastatic disease in this sick patient are obviously very difficult to make. They are based on several factors such as the wishes of the patient and family, the functional status of the patient, the anticipated remaining survival time, the effectiveness of radiotherapy in ameliorating, preventing or delaying symptoms and the consideration of the possible risks or complications of any proposed treatment. My clinical judgement may be based on points of information not detailed in the case presentation but with the information available, I will describe any assumptions necessary to allow discussion of my thought processes in arriving at a treatment decision.

Firstly, my overall impression of this patient is one who is obviously terminal with a short expected survival time. With her major adverse prognostic features being the presence of visceral metastases (mediastinum and liver), greater than three symptomatic bony metastases, and hypercalcemia of malignancy, I would estimate her median survival at 4 or 5 months or less. Her prognosis is not so greatly influenced in this case by the fact that she had an initial disease-free interval of 3 years and later a presumed second interval of 4 years, as I believe the adverse factors I described above are overriding. Some clinicians may believe that her prognosis is much worse than I stated, but my experience has been that similar patients, unless showing a persistently poor Karnofsky status during the first week of their hospital admission, have made sufficient recoveries to return home.

Despite what initially appears to be a patient with a poor functional status, I would evaluate the possible factors responsible for her being bedridden. These etiologies would include a specific myelopathy or neuropathy, pain, hypercalcemia, anemia and other metabolic derangements. Some of these would be more easily treated than others.

In treating this patient, general measures are important and correction of hematologic and metabolic abnormalities should be undertaken. In particular, her hypercalcemia should be medically treated in the usual fashion as this may decrease her pain and weakness. Systemic therapy for her multiple sites of disease and for achieving any durable control of the hypercalcemia has to be considered of prime importance. Unless she is too debilitated, chemotherapy is probably indicated and depending on her tumor receptor status, hormonal therapy may be effective.

A myelopathy causing bilateral leg weakness should be looked for on neurologic examination and

Jonathan Tsao, MD, Department of Radiation Oncology, Southern California Permanente Medical Group, 4950 Sunset Boulevard, Los Angeles, CA 90027, USA

ruled out, if necessary, with an MRI of the spinal column. If she had one, I would start high-dose dexamethasone and only if there was a response would I offer her a course of radiation (2000 cGy in five fractions).

Only after the successful treatment of the hypercalcemia and after judicious use of analgesics would I then consider palliative radiotherapy for the more painful bony metastases. Treatment would be most effective if there were only a few predominant sites that could be irradiated without excessive toxicity to bone marrow. The total volume irradiated would be limited by the amount of prior myelosuppressive chemotherapy. Single fractions of 600–800 cGy to the target volume are sufficient as at least one review suggests that single fractionated doses for bone pain are just as effective as multiple fractions.

In particular, a previous history of Adriamycin administration would probably not otherwise influence my plan, unless a large portion of the heart is included within the treatment portal. However, even in this case, if a few single large fractions, which could lead to acute pericarditis, were avoided, I could argue for proceeding with radiation because the potential radiation and chemotherapy-induced myocarditis would not occur until 6–12 months later in this patient who would not be expected to survive that long. In addition, apart from the potentiation of skin reactions which would probably not be an issue with the use of megavoltage radiotherapy, I am not impressed with any other clinically significant increased organ toxicity with the use of radiation and prior Adriamycin chemotherapy.

I would not treat the mediastinal mass unless symptomatic. Although a Radiation Therapy Oncology Group (RTOG) study showed that effective and safe radiation to the liver with a dose of 2100 cGy in seven fractions could be administered, I would not be inclined to give this as my experience has been that the palliation, specifically the relief of pain, is quite short-lived and that radiation-induced nausea and vomiting can be extreme.

Palliative hemibody irradiation offers the advantage of treating multiple symptomatic and asymptomatic sites of disease. However, I would tend to stay away from this treatment in this patient because of the appreciable side effects such as nausea, vomiting, severe diarrhea, myelosuppression and cytopenias (especially with concomitant chemotherapy), and possible pneumonitis and hepatitis.

8 Palliative Treatment of Cancer of the Pancreas

C.M. Mansfield

Introduction

The American Cancer Society estimated that in 1992 cancer of the pancreas would occur in 28 300 people in the United States and that 25 000 Americans would die from the disease in the same year. The incidence of cancer of the pancreas in 1920 was 3 per 100 000 and has been 9 per 100 000 since 1970. The incidence increases with age, and the median survival is approximately 6 months. The survival is 8% at 1 year and 3% at 5 years. The cancer is rarely discovered early: 90% of patients will have positive regional nodes and 60% – 80% will have liver metastases at the time of diagnosis. The disease is rare in patients aged below 40 years; 90% of the malignancies are ductal cell adenocarcinomas, and 60% of the cancers occur in the head of the pancreas.

Anatomy

The head of the pancreas is adjacent to the liver, pylorus, ascending and descending duodenal loops and is anterior to the aorta, vena cava and the 12th thoracic or 1st lumbar vertebra. The body is adjacent to the posterior wall of the stomach and is anterior to the portal vein. The tail is adjacent to the left kidney, adrenal, spleen and stomach.

The lymphatic drain is into regional nodes that are associated with the major arteries to the gland. The arteries are branches of the splenic artery which anastomosis at several sites with gastroduodenal and superior mesenteric arteries. The superior mesenteric and splenic veins empty into the portal vein. The regional lymphatics that drain the head include the pyloric, posterior pancreaticoduodenal and celiac nodes. The pancreaticolineal, the superior and inferior pancreatic and splenic nodes, drain the body and tail. Other node groups include the retroperitoneal, superior mesenteric, peripancreatic and lateral aortic.

The sympathetic fibers may carry the pain sensation. Pain is probably produced as a result of damage to the nerve fibers, perineural spread of tumor, inflammation of nerve fibers, or spasm of smooth muscle.

Most Common Site and Method of Spread

The head of the pancreas is the most common site (60%–65%), combined sites are the second (21%), followed by the body (13%) and the tail (5%). Spread can be by direct extension, lymphatics, or hematogenous.

Carcinoma in the head of the pancreas can extend into the ampulla, common bile duct, gall bladder, duodenal loop, peritoneum and liver. The extension of a cancer of the head can be into the retroperitoneal space with fixation of vessels posterior to the head. The main pancreatic duct and the common bile duct join in the wall of the duodenum to form the Ampulla of Vater. This helps to explain why 80%–90% of cancers of the head present with jaundice. Tumors of the body will invade the stomach, intestines, mesenteric vessels, and liver. Tumors of the tail extend into the left kidney, left adrenal, stomach, spleen, and peritoneum.

Spread by metastases occurs in 80%–90% of the cases. There are no metastases in approximately 5% of the patients. Lymph nodes are the most common site of metastases. The site of lymph node metastases is dependent on the location of the tumor in the pancreas. Tumors in the head will drain predominately the anterior and posterior pancreaticoduodenal, the superior and inferior pancreatic head groups and celiac nodes. Tumors in the body and tail tend to spread to the superior and inferior pancreatic and pancreaticolineal.

Hematogenesis spread is to the liver, lung, bone, brain, adrenals, and kidneys.

Carl M. Mansfield, MD, ScD, Department of Radiation Oncology, Thomas Jefferson University Hospital, 1020 Walnut Street, Philadelphia, PA 19107–5587, USA

Symptoms

Most patients present with jaundice (80%), pain (70%), and weight loss (90%). Only 10% of patients with body and tail cancer will present with jaundice. Tumors of the body and tail of the pancreas are diagnosed late because of lack of symptoms. Therefore, survival is very poor.

Diagnosis and Staging

Presumptive diagnosis can be made on the basis of symptoms and physical findings or by computed tomography (CT) or magnetic resonance imaging (MRI). Tumor markers may be helpful. For example, 85% will have an elevated carcinoembryonic antigen (CEA) level. In cancer of the pancreas, staging is important because survival depends on size and stage; therefore, it is important to know precisely the extent of disease. A T1 lesion is confined to pancreas, a T2 lesion has invaded into duodenum, bile duct, or peripancreatic tissues, and a T3 has invaded into stomach, spleen, colon, or adjacent large vessels. Stage I patients have a T1 or T2 tumor and have N0M0 disease. Stage II patients are T3 lesions with N0M0 disease. Stage III patients are any T tumor with N1M0 disease, and stage IV patients are any T or N, with M1.

Treatment

Curative

Surgery is the primary method of treating cancer of the pancreas. The curability by surgery is dependent upon the stage of the disease at the time of treatment. Patients with a T1N0 disease of the pancreas will have a high cure rate. Unfortunately, this stage of the disease is rare and is usually found by accident or coincidental to surgery for another condition. There are also a few cases in which the unique location of the tumor causes early symptoms and a resultant early diagnosis. However, although 10%–20% are "resectable," 80%–90% of the patients are stage II, III, or IV when first diagnosed.

For the resectable patient, Whipple in 1935 used a procedure that was later popularized by Brunschwig in the 1940s. Presently, the commonly used procedure consists of a pancreaticojejunostomy, a choledochojejunostomy, and a gastrojejunostomy. The patient may or may not have a postoperative irradiation in the tumor bed, the margins of which can be outlined with surgical clips.

A number of patients after surgery for local disease confined to the pancreas will be found to have microscopic or macroscopic disease at or near the margins at the time of review of the specimen. In others the specimen may show adequate margins with positive nodes. In these patients, the addition of radiation therapy is most important because local control can be increased over surgery alone. Chemotherapy can be used to increase radiosensitization, thereby possibly slightly improving the chances of local control. Several protocols have included the use of combined modality treatment that include postoperative radiation and chemotherapy. A number of agents such as mitomycin C, streptozocin, doxorubicin (Adriamycin), and 5-fluorouracil (5FU) have been used. The most commonly used is 5FU.

Palliation

When it comes to palliation, the old caveat "do no harm" is of paramount importance. The goal of treatment should be to make the patient better or at least feel better. Palliation is not intended to prolong life. If it becomes apparent that this goal is not achievable, the treatment should not be started or discontinued if it is already in progress.

In determining the potential value of palliation it is important to know the factors which will influence outcome, such as the site and extent of disease, what previous treatments have been given, and the performance status of the patient. Previous therapies such as chemotherapy, type of surgery or radiation must be known regardless of the therapeutic modality being planned for palliation. For example, on the basis of these factors chemotherapy can be planned, the surgeon will be able to decide if palliation is warranted and to plan the surgical procedure. For the radiation oncologist, determining the extent, site and previous treatments will help to define the size of the irradiation volume and what normal tissue will be in the treatment volume.

Surgery is the preferred modality in the palliative treatment of cancer of the pancreas. Three major problems that require palliation with carcinoma of the pancreas are biliary obstruction, gastric outlet obstruction, and abdominal pain. Biliary and gastric obstruction essentially require a mechanical resolution and, in this regard, an exploratory laparotomy, gastrojejunostomy and a choledochojejunostomy are necessary to deal with the problem. If a gastric obstruction is not present, a biliary obstruction may also be corrected by nonsurgical methods using a transhepatic catheter passed into the biliary tree for either external drainage or through the region of the obstruction into the duodenum for internal drainage. If anastomotic problems occur at the region of the gastric bypass, a jejunal feeding tube may be necessary.

Cancer of the pancreas is radiosensitive, therefore, radiation therapy has a role to play in the palliative treatment of such patients. When evaluating the patient for radiation therapy, it is necessary to review all of the data available and order additional studies, if needed, in order to obtain a comprehensive understanding of the patient's condition. The combination of radiation therapy and adjuvant chemotherapy may produce the best local response. This potential of response must be balanced against the overall toxic effect of the added chemotherapy. However, on balance it is believed that the benefits of combined therapy outweigh the toxic effects. Nonetheless, these toxic effects must be taken into consideration in the more debilitated or moribund patient.

If the disease is local but inoperable because of local extent, it is possible to cure only a few of these patients. Most patients, who are inoperable because of local extension, are candidates for palliation only. Palliation can be achieved by: (1) local surgery using a bypass or an anastomosis, (2) local surgical debulking and bypass procedures followed by radiation therapy and/or chemotherapy, (3) biliary stents with or without therapy, or (4) radiation therapy and/or chemotherapy.

Chemotherapy, in most instances, is a 5FU-based combination with the addition of leucovorin. A major side effect can be significant diarrhea from the enhanced effect of 5FU, leucovorin, and radiation on the small bowel. 5FU is usually delivered in the first 3–5 days of radiation as an infusion and, if necessary, repeated at the end of 4 weeks.

Approximately 80% of patients will have local operable disease with metastases, local inoperable disease with metastases, or extensive inoperable disease with metastases. For the patient with operable local disease and distant metastases, there is a role for palliative surgical procedures such as the pancreaticojejunostomy, the choledochojejunostomy and the gastrojejunostomy, and depending on their Karnofsky status, they can be given radiation and or chemotherapy. The management of patients with inoperable local disease or extensive regional disease is similar. The first and most important procedure is to palliate symptoms by surgery when possible and to use radiation and or chemotherapy post surgery. In all of these patients, chemotherapy will be the primary mode of management.

Palliation of pancreatic pain requires a multimodal approach. Pain can be severe, affecting the quality of life of the patient. The first step is to provide adequate narcotic medication to overcome the immediate effects of pain. Narcotics and antidepressants should be used liberally for these patients because they are often depressed and have short survivals. The second approach is to obtain tumor shrinkage with active treatment of the cancer by radiation therapy and/or chemotherapy. Following radiation, if pain persists, other options would include a temporary or permanent nerve block, sectioning of the greater and lesser splanchnic nerves and celiac and superior mesenteric ganglionectomy.

Radiation therapy is an important tool in the management of inoperable tumors. Pancreatic adenocarcinoma, contrary to popular belief, is a radiosensitive tumor. Tumor shrinkage, as in other gastrointestinal cancers, tends to be slow and the full benefit of radiation may not be obvious until several weeks or months after the completion of radiation. Patients also require high doses. Responses may be accelerated and more sustained with the use of combined chemotherapy and radiation therapy.

The treatment volume is designed by using treatment planning. The radiation approach utilized is generally to start with parallel opposed anteroposterior/posteroanterior (AP/PA) fields to large tumors to a total dose of 4000–5500 cGy with 225–250 cGy per fraction for stage IV disease. However, if the tumor is localized without evidence of metastasis, a lower dose per fraction of 180–200 cGy and treatment to a higher total dose of 6000–6500 cGy achieves better local control over time. When doses above 4000 cGy are planned to be delivered, a three- or four-field treatment plan and technique must be utilized to avoid excessive dose to the kidneys, stomach, and liver (Fig. 1). Three-dimensional isodose distribution can help to accomplish this goal (Fig. 2).

An additional palliative approach in these patients is to use intra-operative radiation (IORT) or iodine-125 implantation at the time of surgical exploration. It has been observed that pancreatic pain is dramatically reduced after iodine-125 implantation and IORT. The full mechanism of the pain relief is not understood, but clinical observation shows dramatic improvement within 23 h of such treatment in 70% of patients. Iodine-125 implantations usually require the delivery of a minimum peripheral dose of 1200 cGy or the dose that results

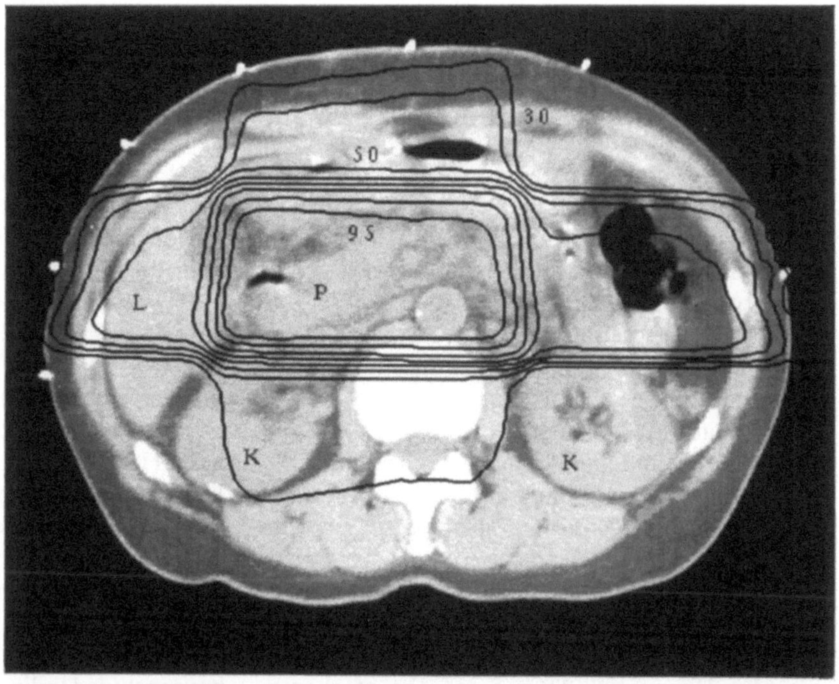

Fig. 1. A four-field treatment plan for a pancreatic tumor that includes the target volume within the 95% isodose liver (*P*, pancreas; *K*, kidney; *L*, liver)

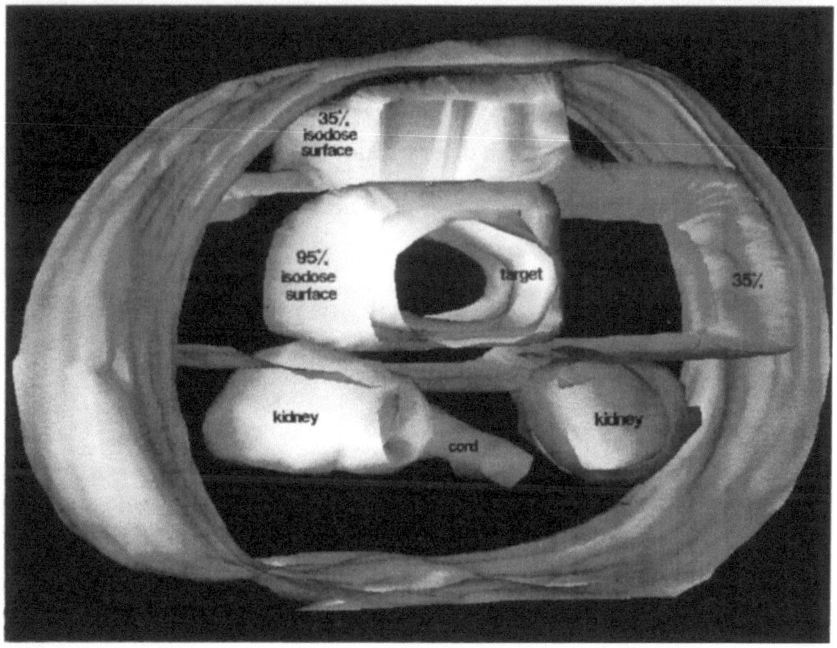

Fig. 2. A three-dimensional treatment plan of Fig. 1 gives better visualization of the target volume on the surrounding normal structures

from the total decay of the isotope. IORT doses range from 1500–2000 cGy as a single dose utilizing electron energies based on the thickness of the tumor.

Radiation therapy can be used for specific problems such as: (1) liver metastases, (2) pain, (3) jaundice and puritis, and (4) brain and bone metastases. Patients with obstructive jaundice need to have their bilirubin reduced because prolonged jaundice impairs liver function and produces cholangitis, liver failure, puritis, anorexia, malabsorption and malnutrition. Reduced bilirubin decreases puritis and may prolong survival. The liver can tolerate a dose of 3000 cGy at 180–200 cGy per fraction. This or an equivalent dosage can produce relief of symptoms such as pain, jaundice and puritis in 70%–80% of patients. The whole liver or a portion of the liver is treated by means of AP/PA portals if the patient has multiple metastases producing liver enlargement. Liver enlargement due to multiple metastases can produce pain, jaundice and or pruritus. Local areas in the liver or porta-hepatis can be irradiated to relieve pain or jaundice caused by obstruction. Treatment for lung metastases is usually confined to an area of bronchial or tracheal obstruction and requires 4000–4500 cGy at 200 Gy per fraction. Treatment for bone metastases is to a local area of the bone by opposed fields to a dose of 3000–4000 cGy at 250–300 Gy per fraction. The brain can be treated to 3000–4000 cGy at 200–300 cGy per fraction with an excellent response of 70%–80%.

A 53-year-old woman presented with gastric outlet obstruction and jaundice (direct bilirubin of 20). At exploratory laparotomy, biopsy of a peritoneal implant revealed adenocarcinoma compatible with a pancreatic primary. Metastases were also seen in the liver, omentum and lymph nodes. A gastrojejunostomy and cholecystojejunostomy were accomplished successfully. She was started on 5FU infusion plus leucovorin. After 5 months of chemotherapy, ascites occurred and the abdominal tumors were noted to be growing. Total parenteral nutrition (TPN) was started, and a nasogastric tube was placed because of small-bowel obstruction. Radiation therapy to the upper abdomen was started but had to be discontinued because of patient deterioration.

I will use this case to highlight the various aspects of pancreatic carcinoma and the role of radiation therapy in the palliative treatment of cancer of the pancreas. Whenever one chooses palliation as the method of treatment there should have been a logical process to reach that conclusion. In other words, a decision to palliate cannot be an isolated decision. There should be full knowledge of the tumor's natural history, routes of spread, prognosis, treatment options and what curative avenues already have been considered.

The most common age for pancreatic cancer is 65–80 years and the disease is rare below the age of 40 years. Age 53 is a little early; however, this patient may have been a smoker, had a high fat diet or had exposure to occupational or environmental carcinogens. Heredity does not appear to play a major role. Her presenting symptoms of gastric outlet obstruction and jaundice are common for cancer of the head of the pancreas. About 80% of patients will have this presentation. Exploratory laparotomy is performed to determine extent of disease and to determine if curative surgery can be attempted. Newer options have included iodine-125 implantation or intraoperative irradiation at the time of surgery. In her case the tumor was found to be nonresectable which is the finding in 80%–90% of the patients. This patient had peritoneal implants, a common metastatic site, which makes her not curable by surgery. She has liver metastases, omental and lymph node metastases. The nodes and liver are the number one and two sites of metastases.

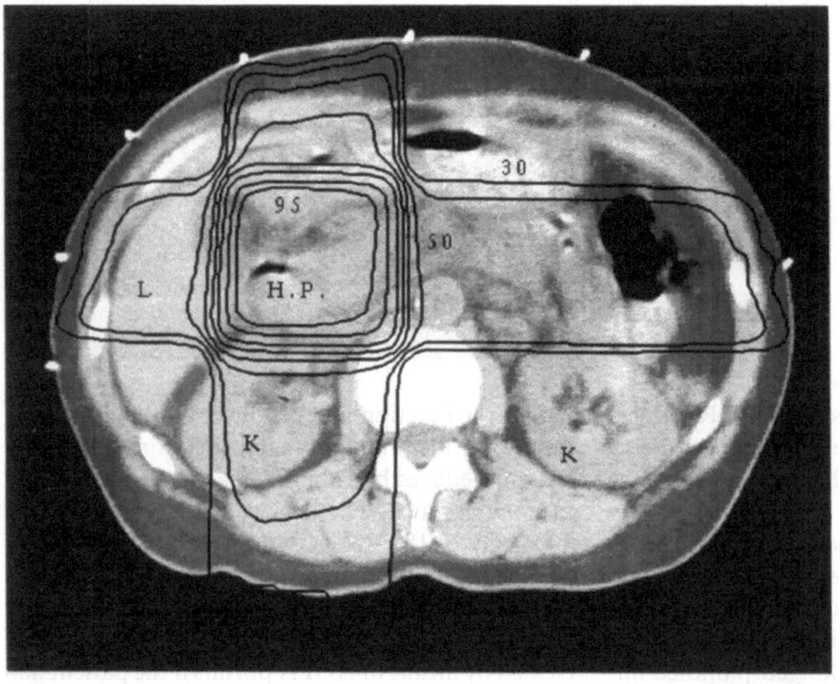

Fig. 3. A two-field treatment plan for palliative treatment of a tumor in the head of the pancreas (*HP*; *P*, pancreas; *K*, kidney; *L*, liver)

In evaluating this patient for radiation therapy it is important to know what palliative surgical procedures have been done. This woman had surgeries that bypassed her biliary (cholecystojejunostomy) and gastric (gastrojejunostomy) obstructions. These procedures carry low morbidity and are very effective palliation for jaundice and gastric obstructions. For the biliary obstructions it is possible to place a biliary stent by endoscopic or percutaneous transhepatic methods. Unfortunately, 70% of stents tend to become occluded in 4–6 months. Radiation of the abdomen for ascites due to pancreatic cancer has been of little to no value. If this patient did not have a peritoneal implant or liver metastases and her lesion was unresectable solely on the basis of biliary and gastric obstruction, the patient would be an excellent candidate for palliative irradiation to decrease pain and provided some degree of local control. Control can be achieved with external beam irradiation directed to the mass. Irradiation can be given in conjunction with 5FU. As noted in this patient, 5FU alone, has not been shown to be very effective but is useful when combined with radiation therapy since there is evidence that 5FU increases the response over that of radiation alone. 5FU with or without leucovorin, can be used in the symptomatic patient. To use 5FU alone or with leucovorin in the asymptomatic patient is probably not justified because of the severe toxicity and little proven benefit. The irradiation technique consists of external beam irradiation to a volume that encompasses the mass and when possible the surrounding local node drainage area (Fig. 3). This volume would be treated to 4600 cGy at 180–200 Gy per day per fraction. If the patient can tolerate further treatment, the field can be decreased to include the mass and treated to an additional 1600 cGy at 200 cGy per fraction to give the tumor 6200 cGy.

Summary

Carcinoma of the pancreas can be treated by radiation to produce good palliative results. These results can be significantly improved when radiation is used in combination with chemotherapy, surgery or both.

9 Recurrent Cervical Cancer with Positive Para-aortic Nodes

H.M. Keys

A 41-year-old black woman had a radical hysterectomy and bilateral pelvic node dissection for a stage IB squamous cell carcinoma. No poor-risk factors were noted on histologic study. Five months later, she had a 7 cm recurrence attached to the vaginal cuff and associated with left hydronephrosis. Periaortic adenopathy was noted on a computed tomography (CT) scan. Within 3 weeks, the pelvic mass had enlarged.

1. Should this pelvic mass be treated? For what reason?
2. What is the prognosis?
3. What dose – time regimen would you use?
4. [Include other considerations that would influence your recommendation].

Response

Good physicians are characterized by the quality of their decision making.

The first decision to be made in any cancer treatment decision process is the most important one; and that is to decide what the goal of the treatment program is to be. For from the goal or goals one can develop various strategies to assess in a risk/benefit type of analysis. This kind of clear thinking is especially important in complex, largely palliative situations such as the one presented here.

The patient is a fairly young, otherwise healthy woman who previously had cervical cancer, FIGO stage IB treated by radical hysterectomy alone, and who subsequently developed pelvic pain and was found to have pelvic lymph node recurrence, and on further evaluation by CT scan to also have gross para- aortic adenopathy. The most important question at this point is whether or not there is any realistic prospect for "cure" which would warrant further evaluation prior to any decision about actual treatment.

Henry M. Keys, MD, Regional Radiation Oncology Program, 47, New Scotland Avenue, Albany, NY 12208, USA

My own judgement and opinion is that there does exist enough hope to proceed with further work-up. Others may argue that I am overly optimistic, and that the chance for "cure" in this situation is less than 5%, and they would have a point. However, I would reason that patients with para-aortic adenopathy at the time of initial presentation have an apparent cure rate of 25% with standard treatment, and possibly higher with more experimental combined modality management. Further, patients with pelvic recurrences after radical hysterectomy do occasionally have their disease controlled or cured with aggressive radiation therapy, perhaps as often as 15% of the time. I have several 5-year survivors in this latter situation in my own practice, one of whom presented with pain and leg edema. The combination of these two recurrence patterns may then have a 5%–10% prospect of cure, which is about the same as a newly diagnosed lung cancer.

On the basis of that reasoning I would proceed with a stepwise evaluation process. First, I would look for any evidence of bone invasion using the CT scan and a bone scan, for I think that bone involvement would dramatically worsen the prognosis without necessarily greatly altering the treatment needed for palliation, a point that I will return to later. Next would be a chest CT scan to look for pulmonary or mediastinal nodal metastases, which if present would render treatment strictly palliative. If none found, a left supraclavicular node biopsy would be done, as I believe that metastasis found there is an indicator of systemic spread and treatment would again be only palliative if supraclavicular disease was found.

However, if none of these investigations proved positive for evidence of incurability, I would proceed more optimistically and evaluate renal function by IV contrast enhanced CT scan (if not already done) and blood urea nitrogen (BUN) and creatinine measurements. If ureteral obstruction is present I would proceed with percutaneous nephrostomy and stent placement to preserve as good renal function as possible. The goals of treatment now become both the attainment of good palliation and local control of the patient's cancer, and attempted cure of the disease altogether.

The treatment program that I would now prescribe is a combination of extended field radiation to the pelvis and the para-aortic disease and cisplatin chemotherapy given weekly during the external beam radiation, and is one that has been in use at Albany Medical College for several years. We have treated 75 patients with extended field radiation with weekly cisplatin. Cisplatin was chosen because it is the single most active chemotherapy drug against both squamous and nonsquamous cervical cancers, and for its radiation sensitizing qualities. Its use weekly is intended to maximize tumor exposure to the combined effect of the two modalities.

Radiation would be given to all treatment fields 5 days a week and cisplatin given Tuesday, Wednesday, or Thursday each week at a dose of 1 mg/kg body weight up to a maximum weekly dose of 60 mg total (an alternative dosing regimen is 40 mg/m^2 body surface area up to a maximum of 70 mg weekly). This is being used in two current Gynecologic Oncology Group (GOG) trials of combined radiation and sensitizing chemotherapy for earlier cervical cancers. The cisplatin can be given as an outpatient infusion with appropriate antiemetic premedications, hydration, and diuresis. Our experience is limited to a maximum of six weekly doses of cisplatin. Not all patients are able to tolerate that much treatment but all of our patients have received at least four doses and most have received five or more cisplatin administrations. White blood cell (WBC) suppression, nausea/anorexia, and severe fatigue are the most common dose limiting toxicities.

Radiation would be delivered to the pelvis at 180 cGy/day using a multiple field arrangement, typically a 4 field "box" technique, to a dose of 5040 cGy. Areas of gross pelvic disease would be boosted to a total dose of 6000–65000 cGy. The para-aortic nodes would be treated a little less aggressively, initially through anteroposterior/posteroanterior (AP/PA) ports, with lateral boost fields used to a total dose of 6000 cGy.

How would I treat those patients who had positive findings on one of the pretreatment studies done to define potentially curable patients?

1. Patients with local bone invasion adjacent to pelvic or para-aortic disease, but no evidence of distant metastases, would be treated in the same fashion as described above.
2. Patients with positive scalene biopsies would be treated similarly with inclusion of the supraclavicular area, as all four of our patients with positive scalene biopsies had supraclavicular recurrences when they did not receive radiation to that area. All four also developed distant metastases and subsequently died.
3. Patients with pulmonary or mediastinal metastases, or those with bone scan evidence of distant metastases, would be treated with systemic chemotherapy and with local irradiation of the disease felt responsible for their pain. This might be a fairly large area in some patients. The treatment course would be kept as short as possible while still attempting to achieve good durable palliation. This will usually mean treatment to 4000–5000 cGy as lower doses are unlikely to achieve this effect.

Patients with recurrent cervical cancer tend to progress fairly rapidly and survival for those who are uncontrolled is usually quite short, rarely as long as a year. Hence, even after the pretreatment evaluation recommended here, one needs to be alert to signs of progression, and be prepared to change treatment strategy and orientation if signs of new disease should surface during treatment.

Part II Preventive or Anticipatory Irradiation

A rose by any other name is just as sweet, and there has been in common English usage for the past few hundred years what the doctor has known as prophylactic, meaning precautionary, medicine. And it would be a slur on the students' intelligence for a surgeon, let us say, to point out, as he has been urged to do, that he wears rubber gloves to "prevent" infecting the patient, gives the anesthetic to "prevent" pain, removes the appendix to "prevent" peritonitis, and so on, ad infinitum. *For his own part, he sits down and has a cup of tea to "prevent" irritation, keeps away from the faculty meeting where the great importance of preventive medicine will again be pointed out to him. Like many, another catchword, "reconstruction," for example, which was on everyone's lips after the War, – "prevention" can be very much overworked. There is only one ultimate and effectual preventive for the maladies to which flesh is heir, and that is death.*

HARVEY CUSHING

Introduction

Anticipating that a metastatic deposit will progress so fast that irreversible damage may be done before palliative treatment can be given forms the basis of many of our justifications for irradiation. The prevention of pathologic fracture, spinal cord compression, postoperative recurrence, brain metastases, and superior vena caval obstruction by irradiation, now rather than later, has often been established by a charismatic oncologist rather than by a scientific method.

After internal fixation, does the entire bone need to be irradiated? Does the use of metamethylacrylate (hyperthermic glue) obviate the need for postoperative irradiation? Should all pathologic fractures be irradiated postoperatively because the soft tissues allegedly are contaminated with malignant cells?

The many definitions of "positive surgical margins" in practice attest to our powers of creative imagination. Do we know how often recurrence does in fact occur relative to each of the many definitions of "positive margins?" What do "positive margins" ultimately mean: local recurrence, distant metastases, both, or none of the above?

With the advent of more sensitive tests for monitoring patients such as single photon emission computed tomography (SPECT), positron emission tomography (PET), magnetic resonance imaging (MRI), prostate-specific antigen (PSA), and the 200 kDa glycoprotein CA125 found as a surface antigen in ovarian cancer, etc, will our desire for more preventive treatment grow despite the lack of test specificity? Does hemibody irradiation or prophylactic vertebral irradiation prevent cord compression, or pathologic fractures in the patient? If the incidence of clinical cord compression or pathologic fracture is 5% of osseous metastatic deposits, how many patients will it take to prove "preventive" irradiation works?

As you the reader peruse the following patient histories, take time to distinguish what we do because we think it works and what we do because we know it works!

10 Extragonadal Choriocarcinoma

A.L. GOLDSON

A 30-year-old white man presented with gyneco mastia over 1 month. The right testicle showed a benign cyst on ultrasound, and a biopsy of the left testicle was normal. The beta-subunit of human chorionic gonadotrophin (β-HCG) was elevated at 5000 IU/ml; therefore, a computed tomography (CT) scan was ordered and showed a 3–4 cm mass at the bifurcation of the aorta. This mass proved to be hemorrhagic choriocarcinoma, and it was successfully removed, with all other retroperitoneal nodes being negative for cancer. No normal lymph node tissue could be discerned accompanying the choriocarcinoma, suggesting that this might be an extra-gonadal primary rather than a metastasis from a subclinical testicular lesion. Postoperatively, the β-HCG dropped to nondetectable levels.

1. Does this patient need any more therapy now?
2. Is there a rationale for irradiating the retroperitoneum?
3. What is the place of radiations in nonseminomas?
4. Are radiations only indicated for chemoresistant disease?
5. [Include other considerations that would influence your recommendations].

Response

Testicular cancer is a relatively rare tumor but one which is the most common among men aged 15–35 years. In the United States in 1989 approximately 5500 men were diagnosed with testicular cancer. Up until two decades ago, testicular cancer was the most common cause of cancer death in this age group. Today testicular cancer is one of the most curable of all cancers with a relative 5-year survival rate in excess of 90% (OZOLS and WILLIAMS 1989). The vast majority of germ cell tumors arise in the testis, although extragonadal presentations arising in midline sites, primarily the mediastinum, retroperitoneum, and occasionally the pineal gland also represent a substantial subset of germ cell tumors.

Seminoma accounts for approximately half of all testicular tumors and occurs in an older age group compared to nonseminomatous tumors. Patient with pure choriocarcinoma represent less than 1% of patients with germ cell cancer. Patients with pure choriocarcinoma represent a major clinical problem since most of these patients present with very high levels of the β-HCG (10 000 IU/ml) and have a higher propensity for hematogenous spread to the lungs, liver, brain and other visceral sites (OZOLS and WILLIAMS 1989).

This 30-year-old white man who presented with one of the common signs, gynecomastia, is an example of the rare cell type, choriocarcinoma. Other signs include testicular mass, adenopathy or abdominal mass. Symptoms include painless testicular mass (50%), back pain, skeletal pain, infertility, breast tenderness and shortness of breath. On the basis of the patient's presenting sign the work-up was orderly. However, the rationale for biopsy of the left testicle was not clear as was the approach taken to secure the biopsy.

Approximately 5%–7% of patients have gynecomastia associated with testicular cancer. The likelihood of gynecomastia is higher with increasing HCG levels. The gynecomastia may be due to increased estrogen production by the tumor, but more likely it is due to increased estradiol production by Leydig cells secondary to HCG stimulation (OZOLS and WILLIAMS 1989).

The diagnostic evaluation of testis cancer should include:

1. Laboratory studies:

   a. Tumor markers, alpha-fetoprotein (AFP), β-HCG, lactate dehydrogenase (LDH)
   b. Routine complete blood count (CBC) with platelet count, renal function tests (including creatinine clearance), liver function tests (LFTs)

Alfred L. Goldson, MD, FACR, Howard University Department of Radiotherapy, 2041 Georgia Avenue, N.W. Washington, DC 20060, USA

2. Staging studies:
   a. Posteroanterior (PA) and lateral chest X-ray
   b. CT of abdomen and lungs
   c. Lymphangiogram (seminoma)
   d. Liver scan if LFTs are increased, and
   e. CT of the brain if pure choriocarcinoma or with central nervous system (CNS) symptoms.

This patient did not have all of the studies indicated, and after the tissue diagnosis was made, a CT of the lungs and brain may still be indicated for baseline evaluation in spite of the β-HCG dropping to nondetectable levels.

The diagnosis of an extragonadal germ cell tumor can be made if: (1) there is a histological diagnosis compatible with germ cell cancer, and (2) there is a normal testicular examination and no evidence of a testicular primary using ultrasound of the testicles.

This patient's history gives no indication that there was palpable abdominal adenopathy or masses, but the findings of gynecomastia, normal testes, and elevated β-HCG were enough to order a CT scan of the abdomen.

The CT demonstrated a 3–4 cm mass at the bifurcation of the aorta. At this point, the decision was made to explore the patient's abdomen. Depending on the relationship between the surgeon and the radiation oncologist, a case like this could have been explored in an intra-operative radiotherapy (IORT) suite to allow for increased treatment options, if necessary.

At exploration, the mass proved to be a hemorrhagic choriocarcinoma that was successfully removed with all retroperitoneal nodes being negative for cancer. All indications were that this was a primary extragonadal choriocarcinoma and not a metastatic process from a subclinical testicular lesion. Postoperatively, the β-HCG dropped to nondectectable levels.

By proposing that this patient could have been explored in an IORT suite (if available) suggests that if the tumor was unresectable or only partially resectable, substantial local treatment could have been initiated without compromising subsequent chemotherapy. Additionally, the IORT dose could have been a preoperative dose especially if the surgeon was concerned that, upon entering the hemorrhagic tumor, there was potential of tumor spillage into the abdomen.

Does This Patient Need Any More Therapy Now?

Answer: yes and no. If the patient is reliable and tumor markers are monitored every 2 months and CT scans of the head, chest and abdomen are performed every 4 months, it would be possible to detect a recurrence and initiate multidrug platinum-based chemotherapy at that point without compromising overall survival (Rorth 1992).

Choriocarcinoma has a predilection to spread hematogenously to the brain, lungs and liver. Therefore, there is a "school of thought" that would routinely start a patient like this on a platinum-based chemotherapy regimen and achieve a 90% cure rate.

Is There a Rationale for Radiating the Retroperitoneum?

Before 1980, adjuvant radiotherapy with a total dose of approximately 40–45 Gy to the para-aortic and ipsilateral pelvic nodes was the standard treatment especially for clinical stage I, nonseminomatous germ cell tumors (NSGCT) in several countries, including Great Britain and Denmark (Rorth 1992). This approach today does not have as many advocates because of the toxicity of this dose of radiation, especially if subsequent chemotherapy is added.

Additionally, although relapse in the retroperitoneum may be reduced by irradiation, the chance of relapse outside of the irradiated field in the brain, liver and lungs is still considerable, especially for choriocarcinoma.

Accordingly, cisplatinum-based chemotherapy protocols have gained greater application because of the systemic coverage and the clinical data that supports its' superior efficacy.

What Is the Place of Radiation in Nonseminomas?

The recent literature is not abundant with data on radiation for NSGCT. Patients with residual masses following systemic chemotherapy would seem like excellent candidates for irradiation, but the literature stresses resection of these residual masses since, similar to primary testicular cancers, the resected masses may contain elements of either residual germ cell tumor, fibrosis, or teratoma. Obviously, if the mass is truly residual germ cell cancer that is not completely resected and deemed chemotherapy resistant, then localized irradiation would be a logical next step.

Is Radiation Only Indicated for Chemoresistant Disease?

If a young patient was unwilling to chance sterility from chemotherapy (cisplatin, etoposide, bleomycin,

PEB) or from retroperitoneal lymph node resection (retrograde ejaculation), a case could be made for irradiation with careful follow-up with tumor markers, and CT scans with the agreement that any sign of recurrence would be treated by multidrug chemotherapy. Current data as it is makes for a difficult recommendation of radiation for NSGCT. An interesting comparison would be of retroperitoneal node dissections plus cisplatinum-based chemotherapy versus retroperitoneal irradiation plus cisplatinum-based chemotherapy. Recommendations to be made after comparing toxicities and survival.

References

Ozols R, Williams S (1989) Testicular cancer. Curr Probl Cancer 13: 285–335

Rorth M (1992) Therapeutic alternatives in clinical stage I nonseminomatous disease. Semin Oncol 19(2): 190–196

11 Mammary Adenocarcinomatosis Complicated by Vertebral Destruction

S.A. Marks

Five years ago, this now 67-year-old woman was treated by excisional biopsy and irradiation for a pT1N0 adenocarcinoma of the left breast.

Three years ago, a left supraclavicular lymph was found to contain metastatic adenocarcinoma, presumed to be from the left breast. She was treated with 6 months of cytoxan, methotrexate and 5-fluorouracil (CMF).

Two years ago, Paget's disease of the right breast was managed by a modified radical mastectomy. The axillary nodes showed no evidence of metastasis.

Constant current debilitating back pain led to a computed tomography (CT) scan of the lumbar spine being performed, which demonstrated destruction of L3 with beginning invasion of the epidural space. Chest radiographs showed multiple lung lesions.

1. What is the role of laminectomy?
2. Under what conditions would you recommend chemotherapy first, for the most current problem, irradiation first, or both together?
3. What would be your planned treatment volume and dose-time prescription?
4. If the internal mammary field had been treated previously, would that influence your current management plan?
5. [Include other considerations that would influence your recommendation].

Response

Breast cancer is a unique malignancy which the medical profession has treated over the years with varying degrees of aggressiveness and yet has still attained little or no improvement in survival stage-for-stage. Only during the recent years have we been able to understand selection of patients for treatment whether they manifest clinically locoregional or frank metastatic disease. Approximately 20% of all breast malignancies are rapidly dividing neoplasms manifesting a short delay in reporting symptoms and carrying approximately five times the risk of node involvement and four times the average risk of occult metastases. Twenty percent comprise the more slowly growing tumors. This type of clinical approach helps the physician select appropriate treatment. At the present time, it behooves us to recognize the prognostic significance of the histological and laboratory methods so that appropriate therapy can be administered when the patient presents with different clinical situations. The state of the art is such that we can now individualize treatment by recognizing prognostic factors influencing the possible length of survival. Breast cancer in its advanced form does show impressive response in certain cases to changes in the hormonal milieu if appropriate modalities are effectively applied. Breast cancer shares with prostatic cancer, a distinction of showing regression following castration or hormonal administration. During the past 15 years, cytotoxic agents have been used with great enthusiasm with the possible exclusion of nontoxic hormonal therapy, unfortunately ignoring the past 50 years of experience with these modalities. If physicians caring for patients with breast malignancy hope to decrease the mortality and morbidity they must reject the view of this disease which has led them to indiscriminate local therapy which resulted in greater morbidity with little benefit. By the same token they must reject indiscriminate systemic therapy which carries some morbidity, especially if proven yield has not occurred. Physicians treating patients with breast malignancy must critically analyze appropriate data. We should not forget the past experiences that have brought adequate responses in breast tumors and only look forward to the hopes of future successes, thereby depriving patients of treatments that have borne the test of time.

In the approach to the management of the case outlined above, we realize that metastatic breast cancer is, at the present time, incurable and the diversity of the relapse patterns are quite unique in this form of malignancy and therefore present an intellectual, as

Stanton A. Marks, MD, Department of Radiation Oncology, Columbia Hospital, 2025 East Newport Avenue, Milwaukee, WI 53211, USA well as a major challenge to the clinical management of these patients. It is important to understand the definition of palliation. This term means the relief of symptoms caused by the neoplasm without causing more symptoms from the treatment that is administered.

A general understanding of distant metastases from cancer of the breast is necessary for appropriate management.

Secondaries to the osseous structures are the most common first site of relapse and are present in approximately 50% of patients when multiple first sites are noted. The second most common site of first relapse is the pulmonary site, which includes lung parenchyma and pleura, and this occurs as the only site in approximately 25% of patients. Central nervous system (CNS) first presentation is very unusual and only occurs in 2%–5% of patients. Of most importance in breast cancer treatment management is the length of the natural history of the individual patient's tumor, and I have personally seen a patient relapse 39 years after the initial therapy and, therefore, one wonders if we ever cure these patients or do they live in symbiosis with their disease. The majority of patients who will develop metastases do so within the first 2–3 years of the original diagnosis. Therefore, we can subset these patients on the basis of their time to the presentation of their first metastases which is important in regard to the aggressiveness of our approach to treatment. The median survival of patients from the time of first manifestation of secondaries varies from approximately 1–2 years with a 5-year survival varying from 5% to 20%, dependent principally upon the age of the patient and the time and site of first metastases. Rarely, a patient may survive 15–20 years after presenting with metastases, particularly patients who had an initial long disease-free interval and respond to hormonal manipulations. The factors that help us determine their survival after manifesting their metastases are patients who initially present with bone metastases without visceral or CNS sites. Patients who present with multiple sites of relapse have a much shorter median survival than those presenting with osseous or a single site.

In evaluating the breast cancer patient with metastases, one has to consider the following factors:

1. Age. Postmenopausal status and, in particular, patients over the age of 70 have a greater chance of long-term survival than premenopausal patients.
2. Initial tumor presentation and disease stage. Patients with large primary tumors, positive node infiltration and, in particular, patients that have more than four positive nodes or present with extracapsular nodal extension or involvement of level 3 nodes, have a worse prognosis. Patients presenting with inflammatory cancer of the breast also have a very poor prognosis even though we are now improving their length of survival to some extent with combined modality therapy.
3. Receptor studies. Patients with positive estrogen receptors (ER) have a longer median survival after recurrent disease than those presenting with estrogen receptor-negative primaries. In some cases, these patients will have a median survival of longer than 2 years, in comparison with the ER-negative group.
4. Progesterone receptors (PR). Patients with positive PR, even with a negative ER, will survive longer, and if they have both positive ER and PR receptors, when they develop metastases they will have a survival of approximately 3 years.
5. Histological type. Patients with special tumors (colloid, adenoid cystic, medullary carcinomas, tubular, and papillary) will usually do better than patients with the more common duct cell and adenocarcinomas.
6. Nuclear grade. Patients with a high nuclear grade have a greater chance of recurrent disease and also have a poor median survival after manifesting metastases.
7. Proliferative rate. DNA flow cytometry for determination of S-phase fraction as well as ploidy status are being used to a greater extent in the last several years to give us some indication of the prognosis. The latest studies are not as enthusiastic using these as a prognostic determinate factor and there is no clear data indicating that patients with a high S-phase and aneuploidy will have a decreased median survival when they manifest metastatic disease than patients with a low S-phase and diploid tumors.
8. Less useful markers. There is not enough data to determine the value of HER-2/*neu* epidermal growth factor receptors and stress response proteins. There is some data indicating that patients with high levels of cathepsin D will have a more unfavorable outlook when they manifest metastatic disease.
9. Timing of initial surgical therapy. There have been some studies indicating the timing of surgery in premenopausal patients will determine the prognosis, but there are no data indicating whether this has any influence on median survival after the patients manifest metastatic disease.

10. Tumor markers. Many markers have been tried in hopes of determining the prognosis of patients with cancer of the breast but none have been very specific and, therefore, are of very little use for determining the prognosis of patients with metastatic breast cancer.

The particular patient to be discussed initially had a neoplasm that was less than 2 cm in diameter and histologically was an adenocarcinoma and she was treated with an excisional biopsy and, I am also assuming that, she has had an axillary node dissection since it is stated as pT1N0. The patient was postmenopausal at age 67. We do not have information in reference to the estrogen or progesterone receptor studies, nor the nuclear grade. She had a 2-year disease-free interval before manifesting an ipsilateral supraclavicular positive lymph node, and this was an indication that the patient had widespread metastatic disease even if we cannot document it on bone scans or other radiographic studies.

It states that she was treated with 6 months of CMF, but there is no indication whether this patient was placed on tamoxifen after chemotherapy. Three years after treatment of the invasive adenocarcinoma of the left breast, the patient manifested Paget's disease of the right breast and was treated with a modified radical mastectomy and the axillary lymph nodes were negative. I do not have information regarding whether a palpable mass was present or whether an invasive malignancy was noted. Approximately 40%–50% of patients with Paget's disease will have an invasive carcinoma and the remainder will have an intraductal carcinoma. The survival is dependent upon a palpable mass, whether there is an invasive carcinoma, and whether lymph nodes are infiltrated. With intraductal carcinoma in Paget's disease, almost 100% of patients will be cured with a mastectomy, and if there is an invasive lesion with a palpable mass, the survival varies in different series from 20%–40% in 5 years, but if there is not a palpable mass and the nodes are negative, the survival is anywhere from 70%–90%. From the case presentation it appears that the patient's metastatic disease is on the basis of the original carcinoma of the left breast.

Oophorectomy or radiation castration is more effective in the premenopausal patient population, and I have noted patients with osseous, soft tissue, or pulmonary metastases responding to these maneuvers. Additive hormonal therapy which, in the past years, was diethyl-stilbestrol (now tamoxifen), is most effective with soft-tissue metastases, somewhat effective in osseous metastases and least effective with visceral secondaries.

Tamoxifen is extremely well-tolerated and there are minimal side effects such as vaginal discharge, flushing, or nausea in less than 5% of patients. I have never had to discontinue this drug because of intolerance, in comparison with the Scottish trial, which indicated that 5% of the patients had the drug discontinued principally due to gastrointestinal side effects.

Cytotoxic therapy, which is principally CMF, CMF plus prednisone (CMFP), or cyclophosphamide, doxorubicin (Adriamycin), and 5-fluorouracil (CAF) is quite well-tolerated by patients, and I would recommend this principally in the premenopausal group of patients whether they have ER and PR-positive or negative neoplasms and would recommend this in the postmenopausal group that are ER-negative or have visceral metastases.

Analysis of prognostic factors should be foremost in deciding on the best therapy. The first conclusion to arrive at is if there is a potential for cure. This is not possible in this patient. Evaluating this patient's course in terms of our initial parameters, it is obvious that this patient presented with stage I disease when all the prognostic factors were in her favor. However, statistically she fell in the 15% of poor prognostic tumors that fail initial therapy and manifest progressive disease. The short disease-free interval, poor response to prior therapy, presence now of multiple sites of bulky disease, are all indicative of poor disease control. The patient, at the time of the second recurrence is a noncurable patient no matter what mode of therapy is selected. The physician has to accept this decision in order to help the interests of his patient, yet has to balance this with realistic hope. The conclusion is supported by the fact that the patient had a very poor and short-lived response to chemotherapy at a time of no documented gross disease. If the patient's tumor did not respond to cytotoxic therapy at a time when there was a very small volume of disease and fewer log kills of cell required, it is unlikely that irradiation is possible now when she has gross bulky diffuse disease. A noncurable patient then becomes a palliative patient. Treatment should be aimed at controlling symptoms, decreasing volume of disease, inhibiting progression of disease, and limiting permanent impairment from the disease with the most nontoxic means.

In the case presented, the finding of most concern would be the invasion of the epidural space. Many patients with breast cancer survive for a number of years and metastases to the spinal canal with extrinsic compression of the spinal cord or metastases to the cauda equina is a common complication and, in particular, breast carcinoma is the most common cause of epidural compression. Physicians have to be alert to the symptomatology of extradural deposits and failure to diagnose this condition at an early date leads to the catastrophe of paralysis with irreversible neurological compromise. The patients initially present with back pain, usually at the site of the level of the extradural deposit and the pain is not relieved by bedrest, as it would be with only osseous metastases. The pain is usually caused by periosteal stretching due to tumor expansion and the radicular pain will be at the level of the involved nerve roots. Once sphincter disturbances occur, the chance of reversing the neurological deficits is markedly decreased with very few of the patients obtaining satisfactory return of function. The clinical suspicion is confirmed in some cases by plain roentgenograms, which reveal collapse of the vertebral bodies at a level of the extradural deposit and destruction of the pedicles. Myelography was a modality that was used in the past and occasionally is necessary, but magnetic resonance imaging (MRI) studies have been much easier for patients to tolerate and appears to be better than CT scanning, since one can evaluate the entire spinal axis. This patient's pulmonary metastases indicates a poor prognosis.

In evaluating this 67-year-old patient, one has to determine the extent of her disease and attempt to determine what length of survival this patient will have. Any patient that is going to be surviving longer than 6 months and has invasion of the epidural space should be treated radically to prevent serious neurological complications. This patient has had an initial 2-year disease-free survival and then developed supraclavicular lymph node metastases indicating systemic disease. I would have treated her with tamoxifen no matter what her receptor studies revealed in place of the CMF that was used. I also would have administered radiotherapy to the left supraclavicular node region to prevent local recurrence.

The Paget's disease of the right breast is probably of no clinical concern since the nodes were negative and the prognosis is excellent with negative adenopathy. I am assuming that there was no palpable mass or evidence of invasive carcinoma and that she presented with intraductal carcinoma.

The patient's present problem is twofold: the lung metastases are an indication of visceral disease and if I had placed the patient on tamoxifen at the time she developed left supraclavicular lymph node, I would discontinue that medication and wait for 2 months, repeating her chest X-rays to see if a withdrawal effect had occurred. If this did not take place, I would then recommend systemic therapy with CMFP.

The findings in the lumbar spine should be evaluated with MRI studies since the detail is greater and also the evaluation of epidural space involvement is more accurate. There is another advantage over a CT scan in that evaluation of a greater length of the spinal canal, epidural space and vertebral bodies can be obtained with that study to rule out multiple epidural metastatic sites. In the past years, patients with epidural disease have immediately been started on dexamethasone and irradiation of the vertebral body and epidural space metastases, but the relief of pain in patients with fairly marked destruction of vertebral bodies having structural loss with decreased height of the bodies had not been entirely satisfactory with external irradiation. Even placing the patients in a brace has not been as satisfactory in comparison to orthopedic procedures. Therefore, it is my recommendation that these patients should be seen by orthopedic surgeons who are capable of performing a vertebrectomy and internal fixation and at the same time they can remove tumor that has extended into the spinal canal. The clinical indications for this procedure and the technical details are as follows:

The treatment of symptomatic spinal metastases remains controversial, with radiation and surgery being the most common modalities. Newer classification systems and treatment protocols have provided new insights. The selection of the type of surgical intervention needed for metastatic carcinoma of the breast depends upon the location of the tumor within the spinal elements, the presence of epidural compression, and the expected longevity of the patient. Historically, laminectomy was the operative procedure of choice in patients presenting with neurological deficits. However, studies have documented that radiation had results equal to laminectomy. Both treatments alone or in combination were only 50% effective in maintaining the patient's ability to walk. The poor response to laminectomy and its resultant decline as a surgical option in the treatment armamentarium of symptomatic metastatic disease has occurred because 70% of lesions involve the anterior vertebral body. It has been well demonstrated that a lumbar laminectomy will not result in adequate decompression and, furthermore, the removal of the posterior elements may increase the instability of the metastatic lesion. Consequently, laminectomy alone is playing a minimal role in the treatment of metastatic disease of the lumbar spine and is presently only indicated when the lesion involves the posterior elements producing symptomatic extradural compression or when there is involvement of multiple vertebrae precluding an anterior procedure. In this situation, posterior stabilization is also indicated. In both of these conditions, radiation therapy would often be tried initially with surgery being utilized for neurological deterioration, incapacitating pain, or segmental instability.

This case presentation involves a patient with L3 vertebral body destruction and the early development of epidural metastases. Unlike laminectomy, more encouraging results with this type of lesion have been noted when the anterior vertebral body was resected and reconstructed. Reports have also demonstrated the superiority of a group of patients treated with vertebral body resections as compared to laminectomy. In most series, 75% of patients who were nonambulatory regained the ability to walk. Radiation therapy continues to remain one of the mainstays of the treatment of metastatic disease and is easily combined with the surgical treatment. In order to provide adequate tissue healing, surgery should be performed at least 2 weeks after the completion of radiation therapy and postoperative radiation should not be performed for at least 2–3 weeks if a bone graft or laminectomy has been the surgical procedure performed. In addition, pseudarthrosis has occurred in patients who had radiation treatment performed at the time of the surgical intervention. Therefore, posterior bone grafting to augment the stabilization has been recommended as a secondary procedure 6 months after radiation therapy. Recent studies have indicated that radiation treatment can be combined with anterior vertebrectomy for which the time interval between the two can be shortened significantly. The recommendation has been a 3–4 week wait between vertebral body resection and radiation. Animal studies have documented bone graft incorporation in spite of the radiation treatment. The role of bone grafting in the majority of these tumors is primarily in patients who have greater than 1 year survival rates – otherwise, methyl methacrylate metal constructs are usually sufficient.

Postoperative management of these patients usually includes the use of a brace. The average length of stay in the hospital is 7–10 days. Early complications from the surgery would be those that are described for the anterior approach to the spine. Late complications would include pseudarthroses and hardware failure.

In the vast majority of metastatic lesions of the spine, the only treatment required is radiation. In those cases in which radiation treatment is not deemed optimal or has failed, surgical intervention is required. Lumbar laminectomy is playing a limited role because of its inability to adequately decompress the canal, the potential to increase the instability of the spine, and the inferior results. Vertebral body resection has provided better pain relief and improved neurological function. Posterior instrumentation is often combined with the anterior procedure to augment the fixation, particularly in those patients with prolonged survival rates. On average, patients who underwent vertebral body resection had at least a 6-month survival rate with a good quality of life. Patients who have expected longevity of less than 3–6 months may not be candidates for extensive anterior vertebrectomy/reconstructions.

Upon healing of the internal fixation procedure postoperative radiotherapy is indicated. If the patient has had bone chips used we should wait a minimum of 2 months before starting radiotherapy so as to allow the chips to become viable, but if the procedure is not performed with bone chips, one can start radiotherapy 3 weeks post surgery.

This patient's prognosis is poor in view of the visceral, as well as osseous, metastases and therefore a fairly rapid course of radiotherapy is indicated. These patients can be treated with a direct posterior field using 60-cobalt, 4 or 6 MEV photons, administering a dosage at 4 cm of 3000 cGy in 10 fractions, or at the most, 3500 cGy at 4 cm in 15 fractions. Another technique is localizing the radiotherapy to the vertebral body and spinal canal region with an open-direct posterior field with lateral wedges using cerrebend blocking devises and the same dosage as noted above is suitable. This approach preserves the posterior soft tissues so that if a second course of therapy is necessary, this can be administered quite safely as long as the total dosage from the first and second course of therapy is not above 5500 cGy tumor dose when treatment is below the level of the spinal cord and 5000 cGy at the spinal cord level. There are certain cases in which an initial higher dose is indicated and those are patients with a long disease-free interval (>7–8 years) who are only manifesting limited multiple sites of osseous metastases with a Karnofsky scale that is 80% or above, and with a patient not having any major system medical problems. In those circumstances I would administer a tumor dose of 4500–5000 cGy. This can be done in 25 fractions over a 5-week period and the patients tolerate it extremely well, but the only technique that should be used would be the three-field isocentric technique with the open posterior field and lateral wedges with cerrebend blocking devices. All fields should be treated daily so that homogenous daily irradiation is taking place and the tissue tolerance will be more satisfactory.

In summation, taking this case as a whole, from the time of initial presentation when a range of treatment options were available from radical surgery, radiation therapy, chemotherapy, and hormonal therapy, the patient has now progressed to the point where her options are limited. This limit is set not so much by the fact that these treatment options are available, but in the framework of the limitations of what should be appropriate therapy. Appropriate therapy is dictated by the natural history of the disease, by the physical and mental condition of the patient, and lastly, by the expected gain. I cannot emphasize enough that the choice should be well considered and is arrived at through mutual honesty and consent between the patient and the physician.

Author's note: I want to thank Steven Robbins, MD, Dept of Orthopedic Surgery for his comments on spinal surgical management.

12 Cord Compression

A.M. El-Mahdi

A 72-year-old man visited a chiropractor for midthoracic back pain. After "alignment" therapy, his back pain worsened and numbness in his lower extremities caused him to enter an emergency room at which time a compression fracture of a T6 with an epidural mass from T5–T7 was discovered. He also had intermittent urinary retention which was attributed to a large prostate gland. A laminectomy at T5 — T6 demonstrated plasma cell myeloma. Postoperatively, he sustained a gastric perforation necessitating a laparotomy. Postoperatively, his leg weakness did not change, his back pain was lessened, his T6 sensory level had disappeared, but he was on nasal O_2 (history of significant chronic obstructive pulmonary disease, COPD).

Laboratory findings which were not available preoperatively were a serum λ light-chain spike, normal renal functions, a serum albumin level of 2.4 g/dl, globulin level of 20 mg/dl and hemoglobin level of 10.9 g/dl and a prostate-specific antigen (PSA) of 55 ng/ml. A radiation oncology consult was requested.

1. Did this patient need a laminectomy?
2. How does the PSA level of 55 influence you? In other words, how important is an elevated PSA to management decisions?
3. When would you irradiate this patient: now or after chemotherapy? Short course or long course or irradiation?
4. Under what situation, if any, would you have recommended orchiectomy? avoided laminectmy?
5. [Include other considerations that would influence your recommendation].

Response

This 72-year-old man presented with an emergent situation: epidural spinal cord compression with no previous history of malignancy. This is not an uncommon situation as up to 37% of these patients have cord compression as a first presentation of malignancy, and the thoracic spine is the most common area of involvement (Flynn and Shipley 1991). The compression fracture of the thoracic spine and the associated epidural mass are certainly common in patients with myeloma but can occur secondary to multiple other primary tumor types as well. Therefore, tissue to both document malignancy and to determine a histologic type for future therapeutic management is necessary. Instead of laminectomy, a needle biopsy of the affected vertebral body, or the soft tissue component, would likely have made the diagnosis. Since myeloma is sensitive to radiation, laminectomy would not have been necessary, nor was it likely to have been more beneficial than radiation alone. Even with malignancies which are less responsive to radiation, laminectomy has shown superior results in terms of functional recovery only under specific circumstances (Barcena et al. 1984; Black 1979; Gilbert et al. 1978). Several retrospective reviews have suggested that surgical decompression should be used as initial therapy in patients who are paraplegic or who have rapidly progressive severe neurological deficit (Barcena et al. 1984; Black 1979; Gilbert et al.1978). If a case was to made for laminectomy in multiple myeloma, it would be under the conditions of a solitary lesion or solitary plasmacytoma of bone because of the expectation of longer survival. A radiographic skeletal survey and iliac crest bone marrow biopsy would help to define this situation. If, however, the patient's diagnosis was multiple myeloma, irradiation could be initiated promptly. Although it has been shown that there is no difference in the rapidity of onset or duration of pain relief between 800 cGy in one fraction as compared to 3000 cGy in ten fractions, the latter is preferred under these circumstances because of the theoretical risk of radiation-induced edema associated with a large single fraction (Rowell and Tobias 1991). For a solitary lesion, the recommended dose is in the 5000 cGy range. The serum protein

Anas M. El-Mahdi, MD, ScD, Department of Radiation Oncology and Biophysics, Eastern Virginia Medical School, 600 Gresham Drive, Norfolk, VA 23507–1999, USA

level and presence of monoclonal gammopathy are of prognostic significance in predicting conversion to myeloma and may provide additional help in the decision regarding dose level (HOLLAND et al. 1992). Additionally, the serum lactate dehydrogenase level, which can be obtained through a simple blood test, is highly predictive of response to chemotherapy and survival in multiple myeloma (DIMOPOULOS 1991). Patients who are expected to have a poor outcome should be treated as expeditiously as possible with palliative intent. Also, corticosteroids are of benefit in reducing neurologic deficit. Although the optimum dose has not been established, the usual dose level is 10 mg dexamethasone intravenously, followed by 4 mg every 6 h.

This case is further complicated by a PSA level in the range of metastatic disease (CHYBOWSKI et al. 1991). Digital rectal examination with prostate ultrasound and biopsy will likely make the diagnosis of prostate cancer, and bone scan will evaluate the potential sites of osseous metastasis. The skeletal survey, which is the study of choice for myeloma, may have shown prostatic osseous lesions as well. Orchiectomy or medical hormonal ablation would likely be beneficial in providing tumor regression and temporary control such that related symptoms are delayed. If the prostate primary is not addressed, it may well become symptomatic and affect the patient's overall condition.

Having taken these initial considerations into account, then, it would seem that there are four different scenarios this case could follow.

1. Solitary plasmacytoma of bone and localized prostate cancer. Laminectomy still would not be necessary if the diagnosis was made by needle biopsy. We would recommend irradiating the involved area of the thoracic spine with an appropriate margin, mindful of field length and spinal cord tolerance, to a dose of 5000 cGy in 25 fractions. Because of the relatively high-dose and curative treatment intent, computed tomography (CT)-guided treatment planning utilizing a posterior wedge-pair field arrangement with a low energy supervoltage accelerator or a 60-cobalt machine would be the preferred treatment technique. In view of the patient's significant history of COPD, a mixed beam using appropriate photon and electron energies could also be used. The prostate would then require a definitive course of radiation as well since both diseases are potentially curable or at least potentially controllable for a lengthy period of time. With regard to systemic therapy, we would suggest observation initially, with chemotherapy reserved for progression to myeloma. With regard to the prostate cancer, the high PSA level would certainly make one suspicious of disease dissemination; however, if evidence is lacking, systemic therapy could be held as well since there is no evidence of improved survival with anticipatory hormonal treatment.
2. Solitary plasmacytoma of bone and disseminated prostate cancer. Under these circumstances we would suggest orchiectomy or luteinizing hormone releasing hormone (LHRH) agonist therapy for control of the prostatic disease component along with aggressive treatment of the plasmacytoma, 5000 cGy as described previously. This patient has the potential for a moderately long survival if the response to hormonal therapy is good, and maintenance of disease control at the thoracic spine would be important to assure continued neurologic function. Of concern would be the potential for epidural spinal cord compression secondary to the prostate primary. Overall, this occurs in 12% of patients with poorly differentiated tumors and 17% of patients who are stage D2 at diagnosis (KUBAN et al. 1986). It is important to recognize the possibility of a second subsequent site of cord compression, and in this particular case from another primary tumor, since early diagnosis and treatment is essential is regaining ambulatory function. A palliative dose of 3000 cGy in ten fractions would be offered under these circumstances.
3. Multiple myeloma and disseminated prostate cancer. The life expectancy with this combination is limited, and generally, the approach should be palliative. The involved area of the thoracic spine should be treated by a relatively short course of radiation, such as 3000 cGy in ten fractions, using a simple technique, such as a single posterior field. The object here is symptomatic relief and restoration of neurologic function. Chemotherapy could be offered for more generalized disease control with regard to myeloma, and the same purpose would be served by orchiectomy for the prostate cancer.
4. Multiple myeloma and localized prostate cancer. The overall outcome here will likely be determined by the myeloma. A short, palliative course of radiation (3000 cGy in ten fractions) can be delivered to the spine followed by chemotherapy. Since the patient, in toto, is unlikely to be cured, the prostate disease, although localized, would be

dealt with, most wisely, by orchiectomy. This would likely keep the disease locally controlled for the typical survival period associated with myeloma. Otherwise, prostate irradiation could be applied should local symptoms develop.

This case, like others found in this collection, presents some of the typical considerations and decisions to be made when dealing with patients who may be in need of palliative as opposed to curative treatment. One must always remember that multiple problems and conditions may exist simultaneously and that to treat the patient most beneficially, we must consider the whole.

References

Barcena A, Lobato RD, Rivas JJ et al. (1984) Spinal metastatic disease: an analysis of factors determining functional prognosis and the choice of treatment. Neurosurgery 15: 820–827

Black P (1979) Spinal metastasis: current status and recommended guidelines for management. Neurosurgery 5: 726–746

Chybowski FM, Larson-Keller JJ, Bergstralh EJ, Oesterling JE (1991) Predicting radionuclide bone scan findings in patients with newly diagnosed, untreated prostate cancer: prostate-specific antigen is superior to all other clinical parameters. J Urol 145: 313–318

Dimopoulos MA (1991) High-serum lactate dehydrogenase level as a marker for drug resistance and short survival in multiple myeloma. Ann Intern Med 115: 931–935

Flynn D, Shipley WU (1991) Management of spinal cord compression secondary to metastatic prostatic carcinoma. Urol Clin North Am 18: 145–152

Gilbert RW, Kim JH, Posner JB (1978) Epidural spinal cord compression from metastatic tumor: diagnosis and treatment. Ann Neurol 3: 40–51

Holland J, Trenkner DA, Wasserman TH et al. (1992) Plasmacytoma: treatment results and conversion to myeloma. Cancer 69: 1513–1517

Kuban DA, El-Mahdi AM, Sigfred SV, et al. (1986) Characteristics of spinal cord compression in adenocarcinoma of prostate. Urology 28: 364–369

Rowell NP, Tobias JS (1991) The role of radiotherapy in the management of multiple myeloma. Blood Rev 5: 84–89

13 Advanced Locoregional Breast Cancer

J. BEDWINEK

A 63-year-old woman lived for 24 months with cancer of the breast. She presented with a mass involving the entire left breast, tethering but not ulcerating the skin and multiple 2–3 cm axillary nodes in association with widespread asymptomatic bone metastases. Biopsy of the breast mass was adenocarcinoma estrogen receptor (ER) positive and progesterone receptor (PR) negative. She underwent chemotherapy with 50% shrinkage of the left breast mass. She then underwent a mastectomy after 6 months of chemotherapy. Treatment with doxorubicin (Adriamycin) was continued postoperatively, and she was placed on mitomycin. After 10 months of Adriamycin she entered the hospital with left ventricular failure, pulmonary edema and a low ejection fraction. Four months before her death, the patient began losing weight and had shortness of breath (SOB) with minor exertion. Her death was thought to be due to a pulmonary embolus.

1. Do primary cancers of the breast ulcerate the skin if left in situ and therefore have to be removed?
2. What is the role of local radiations in palliation of the breast cancer?
3. How do you measure the quality of life in this patient?
4. [Include other considerations that would influence your recommendation].

Response

General Management

The goal in managing metastatic breast cancer should be to keep the patient functioning normally and pursuing her usual lifestyle for as long as possible. Achieving this goal requires a treatment that will cause tumor regression while impacting as little as possible on normal living habits. For this patient tamoxifen fulfills this requirement better than cytotoxic therapy. Cytotoxic therapy as the initial treatment would be justified only if both ER and PR were negative or if visceral disease were present. A computed tomography (CT) scan of the chest extending inferiorly to cover the liver and adrenals would suffice to rule out visceral disease.

The large breast mass and the axillary lymph nodes should temporarily be left in place to serve as easily measurable disease to monitor the effectiveness of the tamoxifen. Since PR was negative, response assessment should probably be done at least monthly in anticipation of a tamoxifen failure. At each follow-up visit, the breast mass and axillary nodes should be measured carefully, and the patient should be questioned about pain and activity level. If the measurable disease regresses or remains unchanged and if no symptoms of bone pain develop, then tamoxifen should be continued. When there is evidence of progression of either the local-regional tumor and/or the bone metastases, then the tamoxifen should be replaced with cytotoxic therapy. In keeping with the goal of impacting as little as possible on lifestyle, I would encourage my medical oncology consultant to start with cyclophosphamide, methotrexate, and 5-fluorouracil (CMF) rather than an Adriamycin-containing regimen.

Local-Regional Management

Now let us address the issue of how to manage the local-regional disease. Axillary nodes, each 2–3 cm in size, and a mass that fills the entire breast create a significant potential for future local-regional problems such as skin ulceration, chest wall pain, brachial plexopathy, and arm edema, all of which can severely impair the quality of life. The goal should be to prevent these problems from occurring, but, again to do so in a way that will impact on lifestyle as little as possible. There are two local-regional management options that could satisfy this goal. One is preventative and the other is anticipatory.

John Bedwinek, MD, Radiation Therapy Department, St. John's Mercy Medical Center, St Louis, MO 63141, USA

Preventative Local-Regional Management

The preventative option is to eradicate the gross local-regional disease, either by high-dose irradiation (6500–7000 cGy) or by surgery (total mastectomy and low axillary dissection). I strongly prefer the surgical option for the following reasons: (1) it is simpler and quicker than irradiation (less interference with lifestyle); (2) it does not produce the intense fibrosis and arm edema that would likely result from delivering 6500–7000 cGy to the entire breast and axilla; and (3) surgery would be much more successful than irradiation in eradicating the large amount of local-regional tumor present in this patient. The ideal time for the surgery would be when there has been sufficient tumor regression to obviate the need for skin grafting. The rationale behind the surgical preventative approach is that, in removing the gross disease from the local-regional area, there is a high probability that the patient will die from distant metastases before the microscopic disease remaining after surgery can grow large enough to cause any of the above-noted local-regional problems. With this rationale, there should be no role for postoperative irradiation. To irradiate residual microscopic disease in the local-regional area while macroscopic distant disease exists is somewhat illogical and represents local-regional overkill.

Anticipatory Local-Regional Management

The other local-regional management option, the anticipatory option, would be to do nothing with the breast mass and axillary nodes until they begin to cause symptoms. The rationale behind this approach is that local-regional symptoms may never develop, and, if they do, they can be effectively palliated at that time.

Preventative Versus Anticipatory

Whether the management of the local-regional disease is by the preventative option or the anticipatory option should depend on the clinical situation. Factors that would make one favor the preventative option are: (1) desire on the part of the patient to be rid of the local-regional tumor, (2) good medical condition such that surgery and general anesthesia would carry minimum risk and morbidity, (3) sufficient tumor regression to allow surgical extirpation of breast and axillary disease without the need for skin grafting, (4) metastases that are well controlled by systemic therapy (tamoxifen or cytotoxics), and (5) poor patient compliance so that the close follow-up required for the anticipatory approach may not be feasible. Factors that would incline one to use the anticipatory option are: (1) patient indifference regarding removal of local-regional tumor, (2) poor medical condition, (3) local-regional disease remaining so large that removal would entail major skin grafting, (4) evidence that distant disease may be progressing, and (5) good patient compliance so that local-regional symptoms can be detected when they are minimal. Unfortunately, it is rare for all factors to be in one direction. Usually there are mixed indications and, in that circumstance, priorities need to be established. For instance, a patient's desire to be rid of the tumor that she can see and feel may override the consideration that major skin grafting will be necessary or that her distant disease may be progressing.

I should state at this point that I favor the surgical preventative option over the anticipatory approach, provided that the surgery can be done with minimal morbidity and provided that the distant disease is relatively stable. The reason for this preference is that observing the local-regional disease until it causes symptoms can occasionally result in a situation in which the patient is too debilitated from distant disease or chemotherapy to undergo effective local-regional palliation. She will then have severe local-regional symptoms to contend with in addition to her many other problems, thereby greatly intensifying her morbidity.

If the Anticipatory Option Leads to Symptoms

Despite my preference for the preventative approach, there are factors, as noted above, that may make observation the superior option. If this approach is taken and the patient develops symptoms, then the treatment of choice at that point is irradiation. The total dose and fractionation of the irradiation should depend upon the patient's overall condition. If her metastatic disease is still limited to bone and seems to be relatively stable, then it would be reasonable to use conventional fractionation to 5000 cGy followed by appropriate boosting of gross disease up to 6000–6600 cGy. If, on the other hand, the patient has progressive distant disease and/or is in poor medical condition, then the local-regional irradiation should be shorter, such as 2500 cGy in ten fractions, or 2000 cGy in five fractions.

Summary and General Philosophy

The guiding philosophy in managing metastatic breast cancer (or any metastatic cancer for that matter) should not be just prolongation of life, but rather prolongation of a life that has meaning, enjoyment, and dignity. Our treatments should, therefore, have as little negative impact as possible on normal lifestyle. Quality of life is as important, and frequently more important, than quantity of life. It is one of the most crucial considerations in making clinical palliative decisions, and yet it is very difficult to define or measure. One method of measuring quality of life is to ask the question: to what degree can the patient participate in life? How much of her day is taken up with sleep, pain, or tending to her illness, as opposed to interacting with family, engaging in enjoyable activities, or carrying out what, for her, are normal daily functions? Asking this question is one method of assessing quality of life, but it should not be the sole guideline for clinical decision making. Quality of life is a much more complex issue and varies from patient to patient. Appropriate palliative judgements can be made only by having a thorough knowledge of the patient's personality, goals, values, and pleasures. Knowledge of this sort comes by taking the time to develop a close and personal patient-physician relationship.

14 Abnormal Cerebral Computed Tomography Scan Status Post Lung Cancer

H.D. KERMAN

Patient is a 69-year-old white man who 3 years ago had a right upper lobectomy for squamous cell carcinoma of the lung with no positive nodes, mediastinal or hilar. On admission currently, he complains of headaches and ataxia of 2 weeks' duration. A computed tomography (CT) scan showed a low-density lesion in the medial aspect of the left cerebellar hemisphere with circumferential contrast enhancement. Chest X-rays, as well as numerous other tests are normal.

1. How common are solitary cerebellar metastases from lung cancer?
2. Would your recommendations change with different disease-free intervals?
3. Would you treat without a histological diagnosis?
4. What radiation dose would you give?
5. If you saw this patient post craniotomy, what is the evidence that irradiation would be beneficial over and above metastatectomy?
6. If abnormal tissue removed from the cerebellum were labelled as hemorrhagic with no evidence of tumor, would you still think of metastasis?
7. [Include other considerations that would influence your recommendation].

Response

Overview

Brain metastasis is a relatively common, and usually fatal consequence affecting patients with non-small-cell lung cancer.

The incidence of clinically diagnosed intracranial metastasis approaches 25% (NEWMAN and HANSEN 1974; KOMAKI et al.1983; FIGLIN et al. 1988), and is found more frequently in post mortem studies (RICHARD and MCKISSOCK 1963; STOIER 1965). Median survival of untreated patients is tragically very short, usually not more than 1 month and only prolonged to a 3–6 month survival in those patients receiving corticosteroids and radiation (CAIRRER et al. 1980).Nonsquamous cancers are more at risk for the development of cerebral metastasis than those with squamous histopathology, and the brain is one of the most frequently involved sites of isolated first recurrences (FIGLIN et al. 1988). Of those patients with cerebral metastasis from non-small-cell lung cancer, approximately half have a solitary first recurrence metastasis, and a fewer number as the only metastatic site (PICKREN et al. 1981; POSNER 1977). These patients are usually best managed by local surgical extirpation with or without postoperative radiation (PATCHELL et al. 1990; POSNER 1990). The definitive role of radiation and radiation dosage schedules is evolving and is as yet not well established. Patients with the initial clinical presentation of a single brain metastasis and a resectable lung tumor are now being considered for surgical resection of both.

Discussion

In considering recommendations for this patient, we are first concerned with establishing both a definite diagnosis of a solitary lesion and specifically that of metastatic cancer. The 3-year disease-free interval following surgical removal of a squamous cell cancer of the lung brings into sharp focus the possibility of nonmetastatic disease, i.e., brain abscess, hemorrhage, infarct, or a primary intracranial tumor. The probability of a metastatic lesion given the CT scan findings is high, but in this instance a recommendation for a magnetic resonance imaging (MRI) study should be made for several reasons. An MRI may be more sensitive that CT scans in demonstrating multiple small, peripheral lesions. Better imaging of the posterior fossa is possible (YOUNG et al. 1981) to evaluate extent of involvement as well as evaluation of the upper spinal cord. Spinal cord failure is

H.D. Kerman, MD, Regional Oncology Center, Halifax Medical Center, Clyde Morris Boulevard, P.O. Box 2830, Daytona Beach, FL 32115–2830, USA

reported to be significant in posterior fossa lesions (DOSERETZ et al. 1980). It is doubtful, however, that differentiation of metastasis from hemorrhage, infarct, or abscess could be made as the sensitivity of MRI in this situation is not enhanced. We would recommend that the patient be placed on corticosteroids (4 mg dexamethasone, Decadron, every 6 h) to evaluate and modulate his symptoms and proceed with the expensive, but appropriate MRI study.

Assuming that the MRI did not reveal multiple lesions and that the spinal cord was not involved, this patient would have the usual, and sanguine circumstance of being the ideal candidate for an aggressive approach to management with the intent of long-term control. Craniotomy would then be offered as the best option for removal of the cerebellar focus, as well as establishing a histologic diagnosis. The alternative of radiation, preferably stereotactic radiosurgery given the location of this lesion, might be considered if craniotomy was refused or if the neurosurgical consultant felt that a craniotomy would result in an unacceptable neurologic deficit.

If the MRI revealed multiple deposits, local palliative radiation to the cerebellum and continued corticosteroids might offer some symptomatic relief. The alternative of whole brain radiation with a short, intensive course with or without a boost to the cerebellar lesion, would also be considered with the intent of increasing survival and a symptom-free interval.

Should there be uncertainty of spinal cord involvement, a lumbar puncture and examination of the cerebrospinal fluid (CSF) might be suggested. Spinal cord and leptomeningeal involvement carries such a dismal prognosis that, if present, further thoughts of aggressive treatment should be abandoned.

We seek histopathologic diagnosis in almost all instances, but it is not a mandatory requirement for treatment. Given a scenario in which the probability of metastatic disease is high, i.e., in this case if the disease-free interval from initial lung surgery was less than one year and the patient had a low Karnofsky functional status score, or if craniotomy was refused, we would feel comfortable in proceeding with external beam treatment without biopsy. With this scenario, the recommendation for craniotomy would be replaced by external beam radiation, either whole brain with a local boost to the symptom-producing cerebellar lesion or stereotactic radiation. The probability of relief of cerebellar dysfunction, however, would not be as great as with surgery.

Following craniotomy, one of two circumstances would occur. The first instance would be consideration for further adjuvant radiation if total removal of the metastatic tumor was successful. Given the relatively long disease-free interval of 3 years, no evidence of systemic disease or multiple brain metastases and the squamous histology, I would be content to recommend that the patient be followed without postoperative radiation. In the second instance, if only subtotal removal of the cerebellar metastasis could be accomplished, a recommendation for postoperative adjunct radiation would be made.

Treatment technique alternatives currently under clinical trial include concurrent brachytherapy radiation with a high-dose afterloading device (T. YAEGER, G. TWEED, and T. BOUTLER, personal communication), interstitial implantation (PRADOS et al. 1989), or noninvasive radiosurgery (LOEFLLER et al. 1990). Awareness of these options, which are current clinical trial opportunities, and their referral sites, if not available inhouse, is the responsibility of all radiation oncologists who are called upon to render management recommendations. Clinical trial recommendation for patients and their families, however, is a consideration which has very serious economic, social and personal consequences, all of which the physician making this recommendation should consider carefully. In this patient, if subtotal removal had occurred, we would probably opt for adjunct stereotactic radiosurgery as it is available in our area as a first choice option given the anatomic location of the tumor. Metastases to the brain from lung tend to be well-circumscribed masses lending themselves more easily to extirpation surgically as well as being discretely spherical for optimum localization and dose distribution for radiotherapy. This would be particularly favorable for noninvasive stereotactic radiosurgery applied to the lesion in the cerebellum. If stereotactic radiation was unavailable, we would prefer local radiation to 4500 cGy at 180 fractions using a posterior arc technique.

Postoperative whole brain radiation, with or without a local boost, following craniotomy has been the usual adjuvant to surgical resection of solitary metastasis even though its effectiveness has been questioned. Survival benefit and neurologic failures have been reported as less likely to occur in two retrospective studies, (SMALLEY et al. 1987; DEANGELIS et al. 1989) but await confirmation by a randomized intergroup trial (Radiation Therapy Oncology Group, RTOG, 90–21) that is currently being conducted.

Brain radiation is not without serious side effects and complications. Neurotoxicity of some degree occurs in about one-half of all patients treated with whole brain radiation to dose levels of 4000–5000 cGy; 5%–10% have neurologic complications which are either life-threatening or require institutional care. Total dose and dose fractionation constitute critical parameters. In general, total doses of 4500–5000 cGy and dose fractions of 180–200 cGy are better tolerated than higher total dose or larger fractions. For short-term symptom palliation, large dose fractions up to and including 400 cGy in five fractions not to exceed 2000 cGy have been utilized without serious difficulty, but if prolonged survival occurs neurotoxicity will often be experienced.

There are no significant data published that chemotherapy, either with single or combination drugs, offers any benefit to patients with non-small-cell lung cancer who experienced a solitary metastasis to the brain. We would consider its use to be inappropriate in this clinical setting.

References

Cairrer Ross JG, Kim JH, Posner JB (1980) Radiation therapy for brain metastasis. Ann Neurol 7: 529–541

DeAngelis LM, Maudell LR, Thaler HT, Kimmel MD, Galicich JH, Fuks Z, Posner JB (1989) The role of radiotherapy after resection of single brain metastases. Neurosurgery 39: 789–796

Doseretz DE, Beitzer, Russel AH, Wang CC (1980) Management of solitary metastasis to the brain: the role of elective brain radiation following complete surgical resection. Int J Radiat Oncol Biol Phys 6: 1727–1730

Figlin RA, Piantadosi S, Feld R (1988) The lung cancer study group: intracranial recurrence of carcinoma after complete surgical resection of stage I, II, and III non-small-cell lung cancer. N Engl J Med 318: 1300–1305

Komaki R, Cox JD, Stark R (1983) Frequency of brain metastasis in adenocarcinoma and large cell carcinoma of the lung: correlation with survival. Int J Radiat Oncol Biol Phys 9: 1467–1470

Loefller JS, Kooy PYW, Fine HA, Cheng CW, Mannarino EG, Tsai JS, Alexander E (1990) The treatment of recurrent brain metastasis with stereotactic radiosurgery. J Clin Oncol 8: 576–582

Newman SJ, Hansen HH (1974) Frequency, diagnosis and treatment of brain metastasis in 247 consecutive patients with bronchogenic carcinoma. Cancer 33: 492–496

Patchell RA, Tibbs PA, Walsh JW, Dempsey RJ, Maruyma Y, Pryscio RJ, Markesby WR, MacDonald JS, Young B (1990) A randomized trial of surgery in the treatment of single metastasis to the brain. N Engl J Med 332: 494–500

Pickren JW, Lopez G, Tsukuda Y, Lane WW (1981) Brain metastasis: an autopsy study. Cancer Treat Symp 2: 295–313

Posner JB (1977) Management of central nervous system metastasis. Semin Oncol 4: 81–91

Posner JB (1990) Surgery for brain metastasis. N Engl J Med 322: 544–545 (editorial)

Prados M, Leibel S, Barnet CM et al. (1989) Interstitial brachytherapy for metastatic brain tumors. Cancer 63: 657–660

Richard P, McKissock W (1963) Intracranial metastasis. Br Med J 41: 19–36

Smalley SR, Schrag MF, Laws ER, OFallon JR (1987) Adjuvant radiation therapy after surgical resection of solitary brain metastasis: association with pattern of failure and survival. Int J Radiat Oncol Biol Phys 13: 1611–1616

Stoier M (1965) Metastatic tumor of the brain. Acta Neurol Scand 41: 19–36

Young IR, Barl M, Clarke GJ (1981) Magnetic resonance properties of hydrogen: imaging of the posterior fossa. AJR 137: 895–901

15 Positive Prostate Biopsy Post Irradiation

T.J. Brickner

A 71-year-old white man was irradiated 7 years ago for a well-differentiated B1 adenocarcinoma (according to Gleason histopathologic grading: 3 of 10) of the prostate. His pelvic nodes received 5000 cGy in 25 fractions and his prostate received 6600 cGy in 33 fractions.

He remains asymptomatic but a recent PSA of 8.2 initiated a biopsy which revealed a moderately differentiated adenocarcinoma (according to Gleason histopathologic grading: 6 of 10).

1. Is treatment indicated now?
2. If not, when? Is further study or observation needed?
3. When and under what circumstances would you re-irradiate? and if so, using what technique?
4. Is a radical surgical procedure indicated for recurrence of an irradiated primary?
5. What kind?
6. When is hormonal therapy indicated?
7. [Include other considerations that would influence your recommendation].

Response

The first basic question asked was "Is treatment indicated now?" My answer to that is definitely yes. However, the nature of the treatment and its purpose are not defined with description of the patient being "71-year-old male." This patient warrants an appropriate work-up and evaluation to make a decision as to which is the best course of treatment available for him. This would consist of, first, a complete history with a review of all previous medical records as well, to rule out the presence of disease which would foreshorten his expected life span such as hypertension, known cardiovascular disease, especially with previous cardiac disease, chronic obstructive pulmonary disease, diabetes mellitus, or other chronic or acute diseases. Should there be no indication that the patient's life span is less than average, then we must assume that this patient will live 12 to 15 or more additional years and warrants every effort at long-term control of his disease. At this point it is mandatory to determine if this is a local recurrence confined strictly to the prostate or if this is a manifestation of overall failure of his previous disease with extension outside of the prostate, either in lymph nodes or distantly to bone or viscera. It is difficult to know if this is a local recurrence or possible even a second primary. I would recommend that the work-up include the following items initially:

1. Posteroanterior (PA) and lateral chest X-ray,
2. Careful complete rectal examination, digitally,
3. Prostatic acid phosphatase,
4. Radioisotope bone scan with single positron emission tomography (SPECT) imaging and appropriate plain radiographs of all questionable areas,
5. Ultrasound scan of the prostate,
6. SMA-20, and
7. Computed tomography (CT) scan of the abdomen and pelvis if bone scan is negative.

It might seem initially that such a work-up for recurrence of prostatic cancer is unduly expensive. However, the selection of the proper treatment to give the patient the longest symptom-free life will, in the long run, expend less medical resources than incomplete work-up and inappropriate treatment with further recurring episodes of failure and more additional treatment. It should be noted that the major emphasis is the determination of metastatic disease, and for that reason if there is a question of metastatic disease further work-up may include the use of magnetic resonant imaging or special labelled isotope scanning. In addition, fine-needle aspiration biopsy or open biopsy may be needed. If there are suspicious changes of adenopathy noted on the CT scan, bipedal lymphangiography may be of benefit.

T.J. Brickner, Jr, MD, Natalie Warren Bryant Cancer Center, St. Francis Hospital, 6161 South Yale Avenue, Tulsa, OK 74136, USA

Results of Testing

The purpose of this extensive work-up is to categorize the patient in one of three categories:

1. Local recurrence with definitely demonstrated metastasis to bone, lymph node, or viscera. I would expect a 2:1 probability of this stage.
2. Local recurrence with questionable findings on one or more studies suggesting possible, but not proven, metastatic disease.
3. Local recurrence with no manifestation of extension outside of the prostate or metastatic disease to other portions of the body.

The role of radiation therapy differs according to the clinical status as defined above. There is no question that radiation therapy may well play a role in any one of these three categories of disease. In category 1, with definitive demonstrated metastatic disease to bone or viscera, I would recommend that the patient undergo an immediate hormone manipulation, most likely orchiectomy. To an orchiectomy may be added the use of flutamide if it is felt the removal of the testicles has not adequately suppressed androgen function. Flutamide is a potent antiandrogenic inhibitor and may add to the benefits obtained by orchiectomy. Even though the patient may be asymptomatic at the time, I feel that there is limited but adequate support in the literature to suggest that early hormone manipulation may extend the symptom-free life span and decrease the probability of bone recurrence (Zincke 1991). To this end, I would suggest the use of hormone manipulation at an early stage. If, for any reason, the patient is not able to undergo an orchiectomy or refuses such a procedure, then the use of leuprolide acetate would be considered. Although this is quite expensive, it is a potent inhibitor of gonadotropin secretion and would serve a purpose quite similar to orchiectomy. In conjunction with such hormone manipulation, the role of radiation therapy would be an ongoing one with local radiation therapy directed to sites of bony metastatic disease as they became symptomatic or if they demonstrated on imaging studies a potential for future fracture or other mechanical problems. I would not recommend external radiation or brachytherapy to the prostate itself at this point. I should think the combination of hormone manipulation and perhaps future transurethral resection would maintain an adequate urinary passage with minimal risk of complications. The patient's life span and future will be determined by his systemic manifestations of disease and not by local recurrence. I would see the role of radiation therapy for bony metastasis not controlled by hormone manipulation.

The second category, one with proven locally recurrent disease and questionable, but not definitely proven metastatic disease represents a bit of a quandary. I would, however, recommend to this patient exactly the same treatment protocol as outlined above. I feel that hormone manipulation with local surgery as needed would provide him with good control of his prostatic recurrence and if, indeed, his systemic findings were highly suspicious, that it would be most appropriate to treat as if they were positive. If the patient was reluctant to undergo orchiectomy or take hormone therapy without proof of metastatic disease, then he could be considered in the third group but with some hesitation due to the questionable findings. Perhaps careful follow-up over a period of 3–12 months would resolve the problem of the questionable findings.

The third category of disease, that is, locally recurrent disease after full dose radiation therapy without evidence of distant metastatic disease represents the greatest problem for management and one in which radiation oncology may play its most important role. The optimal treatment for this category of treatment is highly dependent upon the status of the individual patient. Basically, three or four potential treatment programs are available. Radical prostatectomy or cystoprostatectomy can be performed after full-dose radiation therapy with some significant morbidity, but with a rather low mortality rate. If the patient is in good enough health to undergo a major operation which may last as long as 5 h and may involve the loss of l liter of blood, and if he is an active and vigorous individual who wishes to obtain his optimum possibility for long-term survival then he should be seen in consultation by a surgeon with experience in this difficult type of surgery. If the disease is confined to the prostate and the periprostatic tissues are not too badly fibrosed, it is quite possible to perform a radical prostatectomy. The patient must understand that there is a significant chance, 20%–50%, of some degree of incontinence with slow recovery of this function and perhaps permanent incontinence. This treatment, however, will have the best chance of rendering the patient permanently disease-free in the prostatic fossa. The patient then faces the problem of whether or not he is doomed to eventually appear with distant metastatic disease. In most instances, a recurrence in the prostate does portend in two out of three patients, the eventual development of bony metastasis. In this individual patient with such a long time since radiation therapy initially, the patient may, indeed, have a second primary and may have a somewhat lower probability of distant metastatic disease. My recommendation would be in a very healthy individual with a somewhat vigorous lifestyle and a strong interest in maximum life span to consider referral for a radical surgical procedure.

If the patient has cardiac disease or pulmonary disease which makes such a major surgical procedure a high-risk undertaking, then serious consideration can be given to treatment of the local recurrence with interstitial treatment. The Stanford Group has performed treatment with interstitial iodine for such a situation. I would be more inclined to treat with a perineal template to guide an interstitial implant with afterloading iridium ribbons with ultrasound guidance. In this manner, if the patient had relatively small volume of disease, it would be possible to implant that portion of the prostate containing disease and deliver an additional 6000 cGy. The patient must be aware, however, that there is a potential for necrosis of tissue in this area, and the development of significant problems in the urinary tract and in the rectal region. It is quite possible that the patient could progress to a rectoprostaourethral fistula. The management of the after effects of radiation will require intensive follow-up and management. Our experience in patients who have had interstitial implants and developed ulceration of the rectal mucosa has led us to develop a treatment program which gives the highest probability of control of this disease without fistulization. The cornerstone of this program is an absolute commitment to avoid biopsy of the rectal wall. In many instances it has been our opinion that biopsy of inflamed or suspicious looking rectal mucosa overlying the prostate after an interstitial implant has been the primary cause of deep seated infection, especially anaerobic infection, and the eventual development of fistula. With the prevention of biopsy and with careful management of the bowel function, much of this can be prevented. Soft stool with regular bowel movements must be encouraged. Topical steroids may be tried for short courses, but prolonged use is not of benefit. We have found the best treatment for any breakdown in the rectal mucosa to be a combination of treatment with metronidazole for anaerobic infection, and in several instances pentoxifylline has proven useful. If an ulcer developed and deep seated infection appears to be present and not responding well, a temporary diverting colostomy may be required to allow healing. If healing does not occur, this may become a permanent colostomy. Therefore, it is important that the patient realizes going into this situation that there is a significant risk for the development of a fistulous tract which could lead to a colostomy.

The third alternative form of treatment would be, as has been mentioned above for the other forms of disease, hormone manipulation at this point and careful observation with minimal surgery as needed for symptoms. My reticence to depend on hormone manipulation when there is disease in the prostate, but none demonstrated elsewhere, is that with a 10- to 20-year life expectancy for this age group, I am afraid that hormone manipulation will fail to control the local disease for a sufficiently long time.

References

Zincke H (1991) The role of pathologic variables after hormonal treatment after radical prostatectomy for Stage D1 disease. Oncology 5: 129–139

16 Metastatic Lymphoma and Spinal Cord Compression

T.A. BUCHHOLZ and T.W. GRIFFIN

A 46-year-old black woman has been treated for stage IV diffuse mixed cell lymphoma of the right tonsil with cyclophosphamide, Adriamycin (doxorubicin), Oncovin (vincristine) (CHOP), cyclophosphamide, Oncovin, procarbazine, and prednisone (C-MOPP), 1,3-bis-(2-chlorethyl)-1-nitrosourea (BCNU), and methotrexate over a period of 11 years. At age 43 and 45 she was irradiated to the left axillary supraclavicular region and to the right axillary-supraclavicular region, respectively. Six months ago (now age 46) she suffered back pain which was treated with chlorambucil (Leukeran) and steroids subsequent to a negative magnetic resonance imaging (MRI) scan. However, over the last 3 days, the pain has increased. Leg weakness and a high lumbar sensory level and bowel and bladder dysfunction prompted an MRI which showed spinal cord compression at T12–L1, marrow replacement in T12 and a paraspinal mass. While on steroids, which is also aggravating her type II diabetes mellitus, she can wiggle her toes and legs, but she needs a Foley catheter and has not had a bowel movement since her new symptoms appeared. Her back pain is relieved, however, with bed rest and opiates.

1. Is a laminectomy a consideration?
2. What is your experience with steroids for acute central nervous system (CNS) cancer complications in the diabetic?
3. Would you insist on a biopsy of the paraspinal mass before reaching any treatment decision?
4. How and under what circumstances would you irradiate this patient? Does the previous chemotherapy affect spinal cord tolerance to irradiation?
5. Do you have an opinion on bone marrow autotransplantation following chemotherapy in this clinical setting?
6. [Include other considerations that would influence your recommendation].

Thomas A. Buchholz, MD, Thomas W. Griffin, MD, Department of Radiation Oncology, University of Washington Medical Center RC-08, 1959 N.E. Pacific, Seattle, WA 98195, USA

Response

It is estimated that over 500 000 cancer patients per year receive radiation at some point during their treatment course. Of these, over 50% will receive radiation for treatment of metastatic disease. While often considered to be routine by young practitioners of radiation oncology, the treatment of metastatic disease can present some of the most difficult decisions radiation oncologists encounter. Unfortunately, because many training programs spend an inadequate amount of time teaching techniques of metastatic treatment, some residents are trained in a homogeneous approach to a very heterogeneous category of disease. It is only after years of clinical experience that practitioners begin to appreciate the many important considerations which should influence the management of patients with metastatic disease, and begin to realize the therapeutic challenges that this class of patients presents.

The case presentation is an excellent example of the need to individualize the management of patients with metastatic disease. The example provides many interesting issues which need to be explored prior to making a therapeutic decision. For example, when is a diagnostic biopsy necessary for pathological confirmation of recurrent disease? What is the role of a surgical decompression prior to radiation in the treatment of a malignant compression of the spinal cord? How do confounding medical con-ditions, such as diabetes, effect therapeutic options? How do histories of previous treatment with radiation and chemo-therapy influence the acute management of these patients? And finally, what is the role of autologous bone marrow transplantation in the treatment of recurrent non-Hodgkin's lymphoma?

Acute neurological deterioration in a patient with a history of cancer necessitates immediate diagnostic and therapeutic intervention. In this case example, the patient has appropriately undergone a diagnostic MRI scan which confirmed a T12 paraspinus mass with marrow replacement and compression of the spinal cord. At the time of her diagnostic studies, the patient is paraparetic (nonambulatory but without complete loss of motor abilities). Unfortunately, her presentation is not unusual. RATANATHARATHORN and POWERS (1991) estimate that 40% of patients presenting with cord compression will be diagnosed only after they have lost their ability to ambulate.

When confronted with the case in our example, the most immediate requirement of the treating radiation oncologist is that of performing complete history and physical examination. A careful inquiry should be made into the patient's previous history of radiation treatments. Oftentimes, patients receive treatments at more that one institution, and prior to embarking on a radiotherapeutic course, the oncologist must insure that the patient's previous therapies will not overlap with a current treatment field. A quick but thorough review of systems should be performed specifically aimed at evaluating for symptoms of metastatic recurrence in other regions of the body. The time period over which her neurological deficits occurred should be documented to help prognosticate the chance for neurological recovery. A complete peripheral neurological examination should be performed with careful documentation of the patient's motor and sensory deficits. Rectal sphincter tone should be checked with a digital rectal examination. A careful percussion of her spine should be performed to establish that the area of abnormality on her MRI is the same region as her back pain.

Once the history and physical examination are complete, high-dose intravenous corticosteroids should be started and the patient admitted to the hospital to monitor her neurological status and blood glucose levels. We routinely use a 10 mg intravenous dexamethasone bolus followed by a schedule of 4 mg intravenously every 6 h. The patient's history of diabetes necessitates that the blood glucose levels be carefully monitored. Patients on oral hypoglycemics often require a temporary course of insulin while on corticosteroids. Similarly, it is not unusual for insulin-dependent diabetics to require higher dosages of insulin while on corticosteroids. While diabetes does not contraindicate the use of steroid, the patient is at an increased risk for a steroid complication because of her diabetes and, therefore, needs to be carefully monitored.

An immediate question which arises in management of patients with spinal cord compression is whether a surgical laminectomy and decompression of the spinal cord would be of benefit to the patient. This question needs to be answered on an individual case basis. Indications for a laminectomy include: previous radiation to the area of cord compression, vertebral body collapse and instability of the spine, progressive neurological deterioration while on radiation treatment, unknown tissue diagnosis, and tumors with radioresistant histologies in patients with long life expectancies. In this particular case example, laminectomy does not appear to be indicated. Numerous series have retrospectively compared the use of radiation alone to radiation and surgery for the treatment of cord compression due to malignant disease. GILBERT et al. (1987) compared 65 patients treated with laminectomy and radiation to 170 patients treated with radiation alone reported no difference in outcomes between the groups. A subgroup analysis on patients with favorable histologies, such as the one in this case example, again found no clear benefit for the addition of surgery. In patients with more radioresistant tumor histologies, such as non-small-cell lung cancer, prostate cancer, or metastatic sarcoma, consideration of combining radiation with a laminectomy would be appropriate. A recently published series (LANDMANN et al. 1992) suggested that combined treatment with laminectomy and postoperative radiation offers an improved chance for neurological recovery in paraparetic patients with radioresistant histologies.

The risk of a surgical procedure solely for the purpose of providing pathological confirmation of recurrent disease is not warranted in this case example. The patient's history is not unusual for an intermediate grade lymphoma and the clinical evidence supports the diagnosis of recurrent lymphoma. The risks of a surgical laminectomy for metastatic cord compression are significant. BLACK (1979) reported a 9% operative mortality, 12% deterioration of neurological functioning post surgery, and an 11% non-neurological operative complication rate in patients undergoing a debulking laminectomy for metastatic disease. The risks of surgical laminectomy complications are also greater in diabetic patients. While there is little data specifically evaluating complications of tumor-induced cord compression surg-ery in diabetic patients, LAUS et al. (1992) have not-ed a high complication rate in diabetic patients undergoing surgical laminectomy for benign disease. Weighing these risks against the lack of a clearly proven benefit of decompressive laminectomy in patients with lymphoma, it is clear that surgery be reserved only for those rare cases in which tumor progression occurs during or after radiation treatment.

Once the decision is made to treat with radiation alone, the oncologist must decide on the treatment dose and technique. In making this decision it is imperative to consider all of the following factors: the acute neurological condition of the patient; the radiosensitivity of the tumor; the extent of metastatic disease; the patient's overall prognosis; the possible future systemic treatments; and any history of prior treatment to the involved site. In this example, the patient appears to have had a deterioration over a 3-day period and has significant neurological deficits at the time of her cord compression diagnosis. With this history, it is appropriate to begin treatments with fraction sizes greater than 200 cGy. Treatment with high dose per fraction therapy achieves a greater cell kill of tumor compared to conventional fractionation and allows for a more immediate decompression of the spinal cord. RUBIN (1969) has shown that the edema and the overall mass effect in the area of cord compression are decreased by large dose per fraction treatment compared to conventional fraction sizes. The published retrospective series which conclude that radiation alone is equivalent to laminectomy, all employed a large dose per fraction for the first three fractions (GILBERT et al. 1978; BLACK 1979). Interestingly, one of the only series which suggested that laminectomy prior to radiation improves neurological recovery compared to radiation alone did not give high-dose fractions at the start of radiation treatment (LANDMANN et al. 1992).

Again, it is important to realize that metastatic disease is a very heterogenous problem and requires decisions to be made on an individual case basis. While using a high dose per fraction treatment increases the acute tumor cell kill, it also decreases the therapeutic ratio (the ratio of the probability of tumor control to the probability of developing a spinal cord injury). Lymphomas have a much different radiosensitivity than non-small-cell lung cancer or other relatively radioresistant histology. Specifically, a much lower dose per fraction is required to achieve an equivalent tumor cell kill in lymphomas compared to other tumors. Considering all of these factors, it would be appropriate to begin treating the patient on an emergent basis with 3 daily treatment fractions of 300 cGy and then lower the dose per fraction to 200 cGy and continue with 14 additional treatments. This would provide a total dose of 3700 cGy which, in terms of the spinal cord tolerance, would be radiobiologically equivalent to a treatment course of 4000 cGy in 20 fractions. This total dose would be expected to offer of high probability of a complete tumor response within the treatment area with a low probability of late normal tissue toxicity.

Treatment of a cord compression should begin immediately, with a clinical setup if necessary. The patient should be simulated as soon as possible to ensure that the field size, and thus the amount of normal tissue being treated, is minimized. The treatment field should include one vertebral body above and below the areas of involvement as defined by the MRI scan. The cross sectional images of the MRI scan should be carefully reviewed to ensure that the lateral component of the paraspinus mass is included with the treatment field. Hastily set up fields centered around the cord compression can often underdose the most lateral portions of paraspinus masses. During simulation, a lateral film should be taken during simulation to verify the spinal cord depth. For most thoracic spine fields, a weighted posterior and anterior field pair should be used. The weighting of the fields depends upon the depth of the spinal cord and the patient separation at central axis. A 3:1 weighting of the posterior and anterior field is appropriate for the typical patient with a separation of 25 cm and a cord depth of 7 cm from the posterior field. The lateral margins of the field should allow for daily set up changes but be as tight as possible, with contoured customized blocks around the paraspinus component. This allows for the maximal sparing of lung and kidney. This is particularly important in patients in whom a bone marrow transplantation is being considered.

The patient's acute prognosis for neurological recovery is dependent on several factors. Numerous series confirm that the single most important pretreatment factor in determining neurological recovery is ambulatory status. MARAZANO et al. (1991) reported that in nonparalyzed patients undergoing treatment for a spinal cord compression, 49% achieved an improvement in gait with an additional 31% achieving a stabilization of their neurological deficits. This compares to a 10% rate of ambulatory function recovery in patients paralyzed at the initiation of treatment. The good prognostic features of this particular case include the relatively short duration of the patient's neurological compromise and the radiosensitive nature of her tumor. Both BLACK (1979) and RATANATHARATHORN and POWERS (1991) have reported that patients with lymphomas have an increased likelihood of recovering neurological deficits compared to patients with lung cancer or metastatic renal cell carcinomas.

Once the patient has begun her treatments, a complete restaging of her disease needs to be done. This should include a computer tomography scan of the chest, abdomen, and pelvis, a chest X-ray, and blood studies including liver function tests, complete blood count, lactate dehydrogenase, erythrocyte sedimentation rate, and a copper level. Lastly, bilateral iliac crest bone marrow biopsies and aspirates should be performed.

Corticosteroids should be slowly tapered and discontinued as soon as the patient's neurological symptoms and signs have stabilized or improved. As previously mentioned, the patient's history of diabetes makes her at increased risk for a complication of steroid treatment and it is imperative that she be tapered off the steroids as soon as possible. The radiosensitivity of her lymphoma should permit this within a week or two of initiation of treatment. MARTENSON et al. (1985) have suggested that there is a high rate of steroid complications in cord compression patients, and argues that the complication rate is strongly dependent on the length of the steroid course.

Once the acute issues are handled, possible systemic treatments should be considered. Treatment options and prognosis are dependent on the extent of her recurrent disease as determined by restaging studies, and the patient's performance status upon completion of her radiation. Possible treatment options include additional chemotherapy or bone marrow transplantation. Given the patient's previous chemotherapy history, she likely has received near maximal tolerance dosages of doxorubicin (Adriamycin). Adriamycin is the most active chemotherapeutic agent against lymphoma and second-line combination regimens would not be predicted to have a high likelihood of achieving a prolonged disease-free interval. Because of this, high-dose therapy with an autologous bone marrow transplantation should be seriously considered following completion of her radiation. Over 1000 patients have received autotransplantation for lymphomas, and although randomized data comparing its use to conventional chemotherapy is lacking, retrospective institutional experiences have found favorable results in selected patients. If the patient's staging tests indicate that her recurrence is localized and if this component of her disease successfully responds to radiation treatment, then the patient would be predicted to have a favorable outcome with autologous bone marrow transplantation. PHILIP et al. (1987) have noted a 40% 2-years disease-free survival in young age lymphoma patients with disease in complete remission with salvage therapy or with a small residual pretransplant mass. ARMITAGE (1989) recommends the use of bone marrow transplantation when the disease burden is low and before the disease becomes resistant to chemotherapy. Armitage indicates that the optimal patients for transplant are patients under 60 years, patients without major organ dysfunction, and patients in whom conventional chemotherapy is unlikely to cure the disease (ARMITAGE and GALE 1989). Karnofsky performance status is also an important predictor for favorable outcome with transplantation, and prior to a transplant, the patient's postradiation performance status needs to be carefully accessed. A major concern over the use of autotransplantation in our case example is the reported increased toxicity of this therapy in diabetic patients. SCHOUTEN et al. (1990) have noted an increased rate of mortality in diabetic patients undergoing this procedure. This retrospective study included only a small number of patients, so the exact risk of complications has yet to be clearly defined. Weighing the risks and benefits of high-dose therapy with autologous bone marrow transplantation, it appears that if the patient has a meaningful neurological recovery following radiation and if she is found to have limited disease on restaging, then transplantation offers her the greatest probability of prolonged disease-free survival.

This example has raised many interesting questions to which there are no conclusive answers. Most of the treatment recommendations offered in this chapter are based on the clinical experiences of the authors and data from retrospective studies. Because metastatic disease is so heterogenous, there are many important treatment controversies in this class of patients that will never be fully answered in randomized prospective trials. This case provides an excellent example of the need to individualize the approach to metastatic disease on a case-by-case basis. No other aspect of oncology requires a higher degree of insight, clinical experience, and empathetic care on the part of the treating physician.

References

Armitage JO (1989) Bone marrow transplantation in the treatment of patients with lymphoma. Blood 73(7): 1749–1758

Armitage JO, Gale RP (1989) Bone marrow autotransplantation. Am J Med 86: 203–206

Black P (1979) Spinal metastasis: current status and recommended guidelines for management. Neurosurgery 5(6): 726–746

Gilbert RW, Kim JH, Posner JB (1978) Epidural spinal cord compression from metastatic tumor: diagnosis and treatment. Ann Neurol 3: 40–51

Landmann C, Hunig R, Gratzi O (1992) The role of laminectomy in the combined treatment of metastatic spinal cord compression. Int J Radiat Oncol Biol Phys 24: 627–631

Laus M, Pignatti G, Alfonso C, Ferrari D, DeCristofaro R, Giunti A (1992) Complication in the surgical treatment of lumbar stenosis. Chir Organi Mov 77(1): 65–71

Maranzano E, Latini P, Checcaglini F, Ricci S, Panizza BM, Aristei C, Perrucci E, Beneventi S, Corgna E, Tonato M (1991) Radiation therapy in metastatic spinal cord compression: a prospective analysis of 105 consecutive patients. Cancer 67: 1311–1317

Martenson JA, Evans RG, Lie Mr, Ilstrup DM, Dinapoli RP, Ebersold MJ, Earle JD (1985) Treatment outcome and complications in patients treated for malignant epidural spinal cord compression (SCC). J Neurooncol 3: 77–84

Philip T, Armitage JO, Spitzer G, Chauvin F, Jagannath S, Cahn JY, Colombat P, Goldstone AH, Gorin NC, Flesh M, Laporte JP, Maraninchi D, Pico J, Bosly A, Anderson C, Schots R, Biran P, Cabanillas F, Dicke K (1987) High-dose therapy and autologous bone marrow transplantation after failure of conventional chemotherapy in adults with intermediate-grade or high-grade nonHodgkin's lymphoma. N Engl J Med 316: 1493–1498

Ratanatharathorn V, Powers WE (1991) Epidural spinal cord compression from metastatic tumor: diagnosis and guidelines for management. Cancer Treat Rev 18: 55–71

Rubin P (1969) Extradural spinal cord compression by tumor. Radiology 93: 1243–1260

Schouten HC, Maragos D, Vose J, Armitage JO (1990) Diabetes mellitus or an impaired glucose tolerance as a potential complicating factor in patients treated with high-dose therapy and autologous bone marrow transplantation. Bone Marrow Transplant 6: 333–335

17 Palliative Radiation in Metastatic Osteosarcoma

J.R. CASTRO

The patient is an 18-year-old black woman presenting with osteosarcoma arising in the distal femur and metastasizing to the lungs. Multidrug chemotherapy with methotrexate, ifosfamide, and cisplatin for 5 months resulted in an initially good response, although doxorubicin (Adriamycin) had to be discontinued because of cardiac arrhythmia. A wide resection with knee joint replacement was accomplished but there was rather rapid recurrence, both locally in the femur and the lung. The patient had an above-the-knee amputation for the local recurrence and was started on ifosfamide for the pulmonary metastases. During the next 6 months the patient developed left leg paresis and urinary retention associated with an intramedullary metastasis at T11–12. Further data is not provided regarding the response of the pulmonary metastases to ifosfamide, but on physical examination the patient was noted to be cachectic and on nasal oxygen.

Response

At initial glance, radiotherapy in this setting seems to be of limited benefit. Perhaps 45–50 Gy fractionated at 1.8–2.0 Gy per treatment session might be delivered to the intramedullary metastasis in hopes of relieving paresis, or at least preventing further neurological deterioration. This is beneath the levels of irradiation generally accepted as necessary for control of osteosarcoma, even for those arising in vertebrae or in the skull. It has been a truism for many years that osteosarcoma is one of the most resistant lesions for irradiation, and the prevailing view in a patient with metastases has usually been to accept the inevitable and offer only supportive care. Yet, we have all seen anecdotal instances of surprising response to treatment of osteosarcoma with radiotherapy and more recently with chemotherapy (KELLIE et al. 1989). Thus we must evaluate each patient carefully and as a individual, before deciding on the course of therapy. In this young woman, there is considerable hope that we can contribute meaningfully to her care and possibly even to a prolonged remission.

Osteosarcoma is sometimes more responsive to irradiation than generally presumed (BERTOLI et al. 1987; SUIT 1975; WEICHSELBAUM et al. 1983), and when associated with chemotherapy this effect may be augmented. The possibility of improving this patient's neurologic status, therefore, is significant and given her age, fairly aggressive therapy is indicated. If the patient can be returned to ambulatory status, with return of urinary function, this will provide a significant palliation of her disease process. Although only temporary regression of the intramedullary disease is the most likely event, it should be emphasized that long-term control is possible. Even if this does occur, however, relief of neurological deficit and prevention of paraplegia for her remaining life span are entirely worthwhile reasons for instituting radiotherapy.

Planning treatment in this patient must take into account the likelihood of continued chemotherapy, and possible additive effects on spinal cord tolerance. Also, the length of spinal cord irradiated is important in maximizing dose, and therefore treatment must be predicated on the finding that this is an isolated intramedullary lesion, for any chance of reasonable radiation dose and response. Magnetic resonance imaging (MRI) of the spinal cord should be done to exclude multiple cord lesions or a lengthy portion (>12 cm) of affected spinal cord, either of which would preclude significant irradiation.

I would prefer not to begin with several large fractions (>1.8–2.0 Gy per fraction) since avoidance of cord injury is of critical importance, and doses of 3.0–4.0 Gy per fraction may carry a higher risk of spinal cord damage. Although some would suggest a higher total dose than 45–50 Gy to give a greater chance of spinal tumor control, doing so would require accepting the complication of radiation

Joseph R. Castro, MD, Director of Radiation Oncology, Lawrence Berkeley Laboratory, 1 Cyclotron Road, Berkeley, CA 94720, USA

myelitis with paraplegia. I believe this is an unacceptable technique. We should attempt to keep this patient ambulatory and with bowel and bladder control for as long as possible.

A radiation technique to prevent or diminish dose to underlying tissues such as heart or gastrointestinal-intestinal tract should be undertaken so as to avoid further complications from combined chemotherapy and irradiation toxicity of these structures. Wedged field plans, electron beam or charged particle (proton) therapy might be good methods to accomplish this effort (Castro et al. 1989; Nowakowski et al. 1991; Uhl et al. 1992).

Alteration in fractionation has been successfully applied in osteosarcoma but hypofractionated accelerated techniques would not be appropriate for the spinal cord (Lombardii et al. 1992). Twice daily fractionation of 1.15–1.2 Gy per fraction has been successfully used in the brain stem (Lindstadt et al. 1991; Shrieve et al. 1992), but it is not yet clear that such techniques can be safely used in the spine (Lavey et al. 1992). If it is attempted, at least 8 h should elapse between doses, to allow as much time as possible for sublethal damage repair. It may be possible to raise the spinal tumor dose in this manner but I would be hesitant to go beyond 55–60 Gy until further data is accumulated regarding the safety of this technique.

We should also remember that anecdotal instances of multidrug chemotherapy affecting long-term remissions or even cures of metastatic osteosarcoma have been reported (Kellie et al. 1989; Saeter et al. 1991). A number of agents have effectiveness against osteosarcoma and experience is growing with multidrug, non-cross-resistant, combination chemotherapy (Benjamin et al. 1992; Goorin et al. 1985; Goorin and Andersen 1991; Meyer and Malawer 1991; Rosen et al. 1975, 1983; Souhami 1990; Winkler et al. 1984). Such agents as cisplatin, Adriamycin, etoposide, ifosfamide, cyclophosphamide, bleomycin, and methotrexate are available and have effectiveness in osteosarcoma. Solheim's data have suggested that an aggressive approach involving second-line chemotherapy and surgery is indicated for metastatic disease and that such an approach may lead to long-term survival in up to 30% of patients (Solheim et al. 1992).

I believe that continued attempts at combined chemotherapy and radiation treatment should be carried out since several of these agents have not yet been tried in this patient. This will necessitate careful planning to integrate these drugs with the planned radiotherapy. I would particularly strive to avoid use of Adriamycin or dactinomycin because of the potential for combined toxicity. This should be possible since drug combinations utilizing etoposide, cisplatinum, methotrexate and cyclophosphamide exist and are effective (Cassano et al. 1991; Rosen et al. 1983; Saeter et al. 1991; Souhami 1990).

Especially of concern will be possible combined spinal cord toxicity, bone marrow effects and/or cardiac or gastrointestinal toxicity. Any radiation technique which lessens dose to these structures will be valuable. Thus, an attractive potential future treatment of spinal intramedullary tumors is to use charged particles such as protons in an attempt to irradiate the lesion while protecting the adjacent spinal cord as much as possible.

The initial success of using this technique to treat lesions wrapped around the spinal cord has been reported (Castro et al. 1989; Daftari et al. 1991), and while sufficiently accurate techniques do not yet exist for intramedullary spinal cord lesions, new developments in charged particle beam delivery may make this possible in the future. Under development are dynamic conformal scanning techniques (Castro et al. 1992) which would permit even more precise delivery of localized irradiation with protons. Associated with improvements in patient immobilization, 3D treatment planning, and tumor and normal tissue imaging, the possibility may exist in the next few years to safely deliver high doses to very small, irregular targets with precision.

The careful observation of precise dose delivery on normal tissue tolerance, particularly partial organ tolerance, will facilitate this approach. Such studies have been started for some organ sites (Austin-Seymour et al. 1986) and for proton irradiation of brain stem and spinal tracts (Urie, personal communication).

In summary, in view of this patient's status and continuing improvements in therapy of osteosarcoma, vigorous attempts at combined radiotherapy and chemotherapy treatment are warranted.

References

Austin-Seymour MM, Chen GT, Castro JR, Saunders WM, Pitluck S, Woodruff KH, Kessler M (1986) Dose volume histogram analysis of liver radiation tolerance. Int J Radiat Oncol Biol Phys 12: 31–35

Benjamin RS, Chawla SP, Carrasco CH, Raymond AK, Murray JA, Armen T, Patel S, Wallace S, Ayala A, Papadopoulos NE et al. (1992) Preoperative chemotherapy for osteosarcoma with intravenous adriamycin and intra-arterial cisplatinum. Ann Oncol 3(S2): 3–6

Bertoli R, Brady LW, Thomas P (1987) Tumors of the bone. In: Perez CA, Brady LW (eds) Principles and practice of radiation oncology. Lippincott, Philadelphia, pp 1169–1172

Cassano WF, Graham-Pole J, Dickson N (1991) Etoposide, cyclophosphamide, cisplatin, and doxorubicin as neoadjuvant chemotherapy for osteosarcoma. Cancer 68(9): 1899–1902

Castro JR, Collier JM, Petti PL, Nowakowski V, Chen GTY, Lyman JT, Linstadt DE, Gauger G, Gutin P, Decker M, Phillips TL, Baken K (1989) Charged particle radiotherapy for lesions encircling the brain stem or spinal cord. Int J Radiat Oncol Biol Phys 17(3): 477–484

Castro JR, Petti PL, Daftari IK, Collier JM, Renner T, Ludewigt B, Chu W, Pitluck S, Flemine T, Alonso J, Blakely E (1992) Clinical gain from improved beam delivery systems. Radiat Environ Phys 31: 233–240

Daftari I, Petti PL, Collier JM, Castro JR, Pitluck S (1991) Effect of patient motion on dose uncertainty in charged particle irradiation for lesions encircling brain stem or spinal cord. Med Phys 18: 1105–1116

Goorin AM, Abelson HT, Frei E III (1985) Osteosarcoma: fifteen years later. N Engl J Med 313: 1637–1643

Goorin AM, Andersen JW (1991) Experience with multiagent chemotherapy for osteosarcoma. Improved outcome. Clin Orthop 270: 22–28

Kellie SJ, Hutchison RE, Robertson JT, Pratt CB (1989) Successful treatment of a radiation-associated extradural osteosarcoma with chemotherapy in an adolescent girl. Med Pediatr Oncol 17(6): 514–519

Lavey RS, Johnstone AK, Taylor JM, McBride W (1992) The effect of hyperfractionation on spinal cord response to radiation. Int J Radiat Oncol Biol Phys 24: 681–686

Linstadt DE, Edwards M, Prados M, Larson D, Wara W (1991) Hyperfractionated irradiation for adults with brain stem glioma. Int J Radiat Oncol Biol Phys 20: 757–760

Lombardi F, Gandola L, Fossati-Bellani Gianni MC, Rottoli L, Gasparini M (1992) Hypofractionated accelerated radiotherapy in osteogenic sarcoma. Int J Radiat Oncol Biol Phys 24: 761–765

Meyer WH, Malawer MM (1991) Osteosarcoma: clinical features and evolving surgical and chemotherapeutic strategies. Pediatr Clin North Am 38(2): 317–348

Nowakowski V, Castro JR, Petti PL, Collier JM, Daftari I, Ahn D, Gauger G, Gutin P, Linstadt D, Phillips TL (1991) Charged particle radiotherapy of paraspinal tumors. Int J Radiat Oncol Biol Phys 22: 295–303

Rosen G, Tan C, Sanmaneechat A, Beattie Jr EJ, Marcove R, Murphy ML (1975) The rationale for multiple drug chemotherapy in the treatment of osteogenic sarcoma. Cancer 35: 936–945

Rosen G, Marcove RC, Huvos AG et al. (1983) Primary osteogenic sarcoma: eight-year experience with adjuvant chemotherapy. J Cancer Res Clin Oncol [Suppl] 106: 55–67

Saeter G, Alvegard TA, Elomaa I, Stenwig AE, Holmstrom T, Solheim OP (1991) Treatment of osteosarcoma of the extremities with the T10 protocol, with emphasis on the effects of preoperative chemotherapy with single-agent high-dose methotrexate: a Scandinavian sarcoma group study. J Clin Oncol 9(10): 1766–1775

Shrieve DC, Wara W, Edwards M, Sneed P, Prados M, Coegn P, Larson D, Levin V (1992) Hyperfractionated radiation therapy for glioma of the brain stem. Int J Radiat Oncol Biol Phys 24: 599–610

Solheim OP, Saeter G, Elomaa I, Alvegard TA (1992) The treatment of osteosarcoma: present trends. The Scandinavian sarcoma group experience. Ann Oncol 3(2): 7–11

Souhami RL (1990) The management of osteosarcoma in adults. Clin Oncol (R Coll Radiol) 2(2): 102–107

Suit HD (1975) Role of therapeutic radiology in cancer of bone. Cancer 35: 930–945

Uhl V, Castro JR, Knopf K, Phillips TL, Collier JM, Petti PL, Daftari IK (1992) Preliminary results in heavy charged particle irradiation of bone sarcoma. Int J Radiat Oncol Biol Phys 24: 755–759

Weichselbaum RR, Cassady JR, Jaffe N (1983) Radiation therapy in osteosarcoma. In: Jaffe N (ed) Solid tumors in childhood. CRC, Boca Raton pp 183–190

Winkler K, Beron G, Kotz R et al. (1984) Neoadjuvant chemotherapy for osteogenic sarcoma: results of a cooperative German/Austrian study. J Clin Oncol 2: 617–624

18 Myeloma with Disseminated Osseous Metastases

H. Reiter and P. Rubin

A 59-year-old black man with myeloma presented to the emergency room with severe right arm pain not relieved by narcotics. Radiographs showed a lytic lesion of the right humerus. Six months ago at diagnosis, he had a thoracic cord compression with improvement of his lower extremity strength after steroids, melphalan (Alkeran), and irradiation. His medical diagnosis includes glucose-6-phosphate dehydrogenase (G-6-P-D) deficiency, hypertension and bleeding peptic ulcer. Hemoglobin was 12.1 g/l, white blood cells (WBC) 3100 cells/mm^3, blood urea nitrogen (BUN) 14 mmol/l, creatinine 0.9 mg/dl, and calcium 10.1 mg/dl. A bone survey showed disseminated osseous metastases, more pronounced in ribs, skull, and bone of both arms.

1. Besides the painful right arm, how many other sites would you irradiate?
2. What is the role of hemibody irradiation in this disease?
   a. Would you modify it because of the previous thoracic spine irradiation?
   b. Would you treat the lower half of the body electively?
3. Are other chemotherapeutics helpful in patients who have failed on Alkeran and steroids?
4. [Include other considerations that would influence your recommendations].

Introduction

Perhaps nowhere else is the tenuous interrelationship of the science of medicine and the art of medicine so nebulously drawn as in the delivery of palliative care. With the newest, most expensive technology available, the finest and most experienced radiation oncologists enter the therapeutic arena having acknowledged defeat in the fight for a cure. To preserve what we can, we must change the rules of the battle, so that the aim becomes making good on the promise to the patient of "allowing him as good a quality of life as possible for as long as possible." The armamentarium includes making full use of not just technical abilities and training, but humanity displayed in whatever form is most helpful to the patient.

H. Reiter, MD, P. Rubin, MD, University of Rochester Medical Center, 601 Elmwood Avenue, Box 647, Rochester, NY 14642, USA

The Science

Reactive Versus Proactive Therapy

The two reasons to offer a patient radiation as palliation are to control symptoms which are already present, or to avoid/delay impending symptoms. The first decision to make is whether reactive or proactive treatment is to be considered. In the case as presented, one feature is the painful right humerus, which is to be treated. But the patient also has evidence of bone survey of disseminated osseous metastases, more pronounced in ribs, skull, and bones of both arms. The potential for future problems arising at different sites encompasses a wide range of possibilities, each of which must be measured independently to decide upon the appropriateness of therapy offered to avoid or delay that problem.

Grading Potential Problems

If medicine was an ideal science, one would know definitively the mathematical values to answer each of the following:

1. The likelihood of problem x arising in the absence of proactive irradiation.
2. The likelihood of problem x arising in the presence of proactive irradiation.
3. The decrease in the patient's present quality of life which would be caused by problem x. His present quality of life is a vital consideration. The value one would ascribe for the problem "paraplegia

due to cord compression", assuming that he had a complete return to normal neurologic status following his thoracic cord compression, is higher relative to the value ascribed if he had a significant residual neurologic deficit presently.

4. In the absence of proactive irradiation and the subsequent occurrence of problem x, the likelihood of problem x continuing despite the application of reactive irradiation once the presence of that problem has been identified. The inherent assumption made for the sake of simplicity is that the severity of the problem remains the same regardless of whether the irradiation is offered proactively or reactively. Obviously, this is not always the case and must be kept in mind. The neurologic status of our cord compression scenario, for example, may be far worse if the patient were treated reactively.
5. The likelihood of problem y occurring in the absence of proactive irradiation. For simplicity, problem y will represent all of the myriad of potential side effects of irradiation.
6. The likelihood of problem y occurring in the presence of proactive irradiation. Concerns regarding bone marrow suppression using large field irradiation are enhanced by the history of bleeding peptic ulcer. As well, G-6-P-D deficiency raises the question of uric acid levels after treatment to large fields.
7. The decrease in the patient's present quality of life that would be caused by problem y. As indicated above, his present quality of life is a vital consideration.
8. In the absence of proactive irradiation and the subsequent occurrence of problem x, the likelihood of problem y occurring due to reactive irradiation.

Now if medicine were simply a science, the value of proactive irradiation would be easily calculated as:

Benefit of proactive irradiation for problem

$$x=[(1)-(2)\times 4]\times 3$$

The risk of proactive irradiation for problem

$$x=[(6)-(5)\times(8)]\times 7$$

As always, if benefits outweigh the risks, then the proposed treatment is reasonable. If different options for treatment exist, then the treatment (or nontreatment) with the greatest benefits versus risks differential would be recommended.

As an example, if the problem of pathologic fracture of a long bone of the left arm was potentially to be treated by proactive irradiation of that bone, and the values of points 1–8 listed above were known to be: (1) = 40%, (2) = 10%, (3) = 0.5 (on a scale of 0 to 1 with 1 being the most severe), (4) = 0%, (5) = 0%, (6) = 10%, (7) = 0.1 (on a scale of 0 to 1 with 1 being the most severe), (8) = 10%, then the benefits and the risks of that treatment would be 0.2 and 0.01, respectively, and that treatment could be offered. If, on the other hand, upper hemibody irradiation designed to proactively address pathological fracture of long bones of the arms, spinal cord compression, localized pain, or radicular pain, etc., had a better benefits versus risks differential, then that option should be considered more favorable.

The Options

Localized Field Irradiation

The greatest risk for a poorly controlled problem in the future would be pathological fracture of a long bone in an arm. The drawbacks of such a treatment, as suggested above using hypothetical numbers, are minimal. As well, irradiation after fracture is of course useless for avoiding the problem. Such therapy is therefore easy enough to defend if the long bones are at risk.

Upper Hemibody Irradiation

Hemibody irradiation has been utilized for a number of diseases, most commonly for diffusely metastatic breast, prostate and lung cancer and less often for multiple myeloma. In Radiation Therapy Oncology Group (RTOG) trials 74-02 and 78-10 (Salazar et al. 1981, 1986), comparison of results between conventional local field irradiation and hemibody irradiation, respectively, alone suggested equivalence for ultimate combined pain control (measured as a combination of narcotic requirements and pain scale values) if one did not allow for retreatments, but the patients in RTOG 74-02 treated with local field irradiation had a greater likelihood of complete pain control if one did allow for such retreatments. To settle the issue, RTOG 82-06 randomized patients to local field or to local field plus hemibody irradiation with the latter arm showing at least a delay in future problems. Specifically, benefit for that arm included time-to-disease progression at 1 year, new disease at 1 year, and median time-to-new disease (Poulter et al. 1992). After 30 Gy in ten fractions to local field, doses of 8 Gy were prescribed in a single hemibody dose and the lungs were attenuated with lung corrections, to 7 Gy. In our case, however, these data should be applied with caution. There were few multiple myeloma patients among the total of 499 patients randomized, and other studies have shown significant, sometimes life-threatening, toxicity to bone marrow in multiple myeloma patients when hemibody doses in this range are given sequentially with chemotherapy (RUBIN et al. 1985; SALAZAR et al. 1981). The relative radiosensitivity of multiple myeloma tumor cells may allow reduction of the total dose and hence side effects of therapy while still maintaining benefit to the patient. A dose of 6 Gy would certainly be safer, with lower doses to be used if the irradiation is to be given in close conjunction temporally with chemotherapy. The previously irradiated thoracic spinal cord would have to be shielded to maintain an acceptable level of safety. Insufficient data exist to comment upon the advisability of radiosensitizers, radioprotectors, or multiple fraction schedules. While lower hemibody irradiation might also contribute to delay or avoidance of future problems, the chance for such benefit is less than for the upper hemibody, where more pronounced disease is noted on bone survey, and the risk of myelotoxicity rises, so this would not be recommended proactively.

Chemotherapy

In the setting of relapse after Alkeran and steroids, the use of either high-dose intermittent cyclophosphamide (BERGSAGEL et al. 1972) or a combination of vincristine, BCNU, doxorubicin and prednisone (BONNET et al. 1982) in prospective nonrandomized studies have demonstrated responses in 30% of patients. However, myelotoxicity and particularly thrombocytopenia in our patient with peptic ulcer disease is a significant risk if he is to be treated with hemibody irradiation as well. If a myelotoxic chemotherapeutic regimen was being pursued by the patient, it would not be advisable to treat him proactively to large fields. Only where no similarly myelotoxic therapy is to be used should hemibody irradiation be considered.

The Art

The Players

Obviously, the palliative situation does not fit into simple mathematical formulae, and what is in the best interests of the patient is ultimately (and optimally) decided by the patient. But there is a complex interaction between the patient, significant family members and friends, and the health care providers, and often the goals of one do not agree with the goals of another. There is a need for adaptability on the part of the physician to ensure that the wishes of the patient are honored, so long as they are reasonably attainable. While absolute objectivity on the part of the physician is a technical ideal, ultimately it is the art of medicine which is under greatest demand. Anyone with a modicum of understanding of radiotherapy can define specific criteria for treatment, absolute dose specifications, target volume, etc., but something else entirely is often needed to give the patient and significant relatives and friends the comfort that they seek. In the treatment of one woman with metastatic breast cancer with palliative chemotherapy, I would regularly trade insults with her for recreation, a relationship which would hardly be advisable with most patients. I admitted her one day in neutropenic sepsis, and she told me after her recovery that what frightened her most that day was that I had failed to insult her.

How Aggressive?

Hippocrates' admonition of "above all, do no harm" must of necessity be balanced by the willingness to be aggressive in the pursuit of good quality of life in the face of incurable disease. So long as the benefits outweigh the risks, ideally one should be able to offer aggressive therapy. An underlying assumption is that there exists potential for protracted life, a category under which this patient is assumed to fall (ALEXANIAN et al. 1975).

Conclusion

The recommendations for treatment for this gentleman, allowing for patient wishes and influence of family members and friends, would be local field irradiation to the present site of pain, as well as to any long bones of the arms at risk for pathological fracture, to a dose of 30 Gy in ten fractions over 2 weeks. If the patient is being planned for myelotoxic second-line chemotherapy, no further treatment would be offered at this time, but rather reserved for such a time as further radiation would ameliorate new problems. If, however, the patient is not being planned for second-line chemotherapy, upper hemibody irradiation to a dose of 6 Gy in one fraction, or less if his antecedent Alkeran and prednisone has been given recently, would be appropriate, with lung correction and shielding of the previously irradiated thoracic spinal cord.

References

Alexanian R, Balcerzak S, Bonnet JD, Gehan EA, Haut A, Hewlett JS, Monto RW (1975) Prognostic factors in multiple myeloma. Cancer 36: 1192–1201

Bergsagel DE, Cowan DH, Hasselback R (1972) Plasma cell myeloma: response of melphalan-resistant patients to high-dose intermittent cyclophosphamide. CMA J 107: 851–855

Bonnet J, Alexanian R, Salmon S, Bottomley R, Amare M, Haut A, Dixon D (1982) Vincristine, BCNU, doxorubicin, and prednisone (VBAP) combination in the treatment of relapsing or resistant multiple myeloma: a Southwest Oncology Group study. Cancer Treat Rep 66: 1267–1271

Poulter CA, Cosmatos D, Rubin P, Urtasun R, Cooper JS, Kuske RR, Hornback N, Coughlin C, Weigensberg I, Rotman M (1992) A report of RTOG 8206: a phase III study of whether the addition of single-dose hemibody irradiation to standard fractionated local field irradiation is more effective than local field irradiation alone in the treatment of symptomatic osseous metastases. Int J Radiat Oncol Biol Phys 23: 207–214

Rubin P, Salazar O, Zagars G, Constine LS, Keys H, Poulter CA, Van Ess JD (1985) Systemic hemibody irradiation for overt and occult metastases. Cancer 55: 2210–2221[Suppl]

Salazar OM, Rubin P, Hendrickson RT, Poulter C, Zagars G, Feldman MI, Asbell S, Doss L (1981) Single-dose half-body irradiation for the palliative of multiple bone metastases from solid tumors: a preliminary report. Int J Radiat Oncol Biol Phys 7: 773–781

Salazar OM, Rubin P, Hendrickson FR, Komaki R, Poulter C, Newall J, Asbell SO, Mohiuddin M, Van Ess J (1986) Single-dose half-body irradiation for palliation of multiple bone metastases from solid tumors. Cancer 58: 29–36

19 Rising Carcinoembryonic Antigen Levels Two Years After Postoperative Irradiation

T.A. RICH

This 46-year-old woman had a low anterior resection of a grade 1 polypoid adenocarcinoma of the rectum at 10 cm. One of ten nodes was positive. Preoperatively and postoperatively, her level of carcinoembryonic antigen (CEA) was 12 ng/ml. Postoperative irradiation was given.

Two years later her CEA level was 17 ng/ml. A soft density in the upper anterior one-third of the vaginal wall was described on computed tomography (CT) but could not be palpated.

1. Would you recommend a second look laparoscopy on the basis of the rising CEA level?
2. Would you re-irradiate if cancer were found? What technique would you use?
3. Would you put this patient on chemotherapy?
4. [Include other considerations that would influence your recommendation].

Response

A 46-year-old perimenopausal woman presents with a history of having a low rectal cancer at 10 cm. She is treated initially with a low anterior resection. The pathologic evaluation of the tumor specimen shows transmural tumor invasion and one of ten lymph nodes contains metastatic adenocarcinoma (stage T3N1). Laboratory evaluation shows a preoperative CEA measuring 12 ng/ml; a postoperative CEA level taken 2 weeks after the completion of surgery is also 12 ng/ml. The half-life of CEA is 6 days making this elevated postoperative CEA level related either to co-morbid disease or tobacco smoking. Postoperative irradiation using X-ray radiation treatment (XRT) is administered to the pelvis.

Today, the use of combined modality therapy for postoperative treatment for operable rectal cancer in the United States is based on prospective trials showing that both systemic chemotherapy and XRT (chemoradiation) result in better survival than when either alone is given (KROOK et al. 1991). The best sequence of these treatments has not been evaluated. From a technical perspective, the XRT treatment technique should irradiate the entire true pelvis using a bowel-exclusion method (RICH 1986). A dose of 55 Gy administered in 28–30 fractions is used. We recommend currently that patients receive low-dose continuous infusion 5-fluorouracil (5FU) 300 mg/m^2 daily for 5 days/week with each week of XRT treatment. Both XRT and chemotherapy are interrupted on each weekend to ameliorate acute toxicities which can be increased with combined modality treatment when compared to postoperative XRT alone (RICH 1992).

Chemoradiation is not altered because of an elevation of the CEA postoperative level. In over 200 patients treated with postoperative XRT at the University of Texas MD Anderson Cancer Center, very few patients have presented for postoperative XRT with an elevated CEA level. In a single patient, a computed tomography (CT) scan of the abdomen showed liver metastasis which had been clinically undetected at the time of surgical exploration approximately 10 weeks prior to obtaining the elevated CEA level. We interpret an elevated postoperative CEA level of 12 ng/ml to indicate residual disease and would do a CT scan of the abdomen and pelvis and a chest X-ray prior to starting adjuvant pelvic XRT. Patients with demonstrable metastatic disease would not be candidates for XRT in the face of rapidly progressive metastatic disease outside of the pelvis. Patients with measurable disease would be eligible for phase I/II protocols examining the use of newer systemic agents or more standard systemic chemotherapy consisting of 5FU alone or combined with leucovorin.

In a patient with both an elevated CEA and an abnormality on pelvic CT scan we consider this as progressive residual disease. For these patients with rapidly growing pelvic disease, there would be a good argument for using a rapid fractionation

Tyvin A. Rich, MD, Department of Radiotherapy, University of Texas MD , Anderson Cancer Center, 1515 Holcombe Boulevard, Houston, TX 77030, USA

schedule, or accelerated treatment, in order to achieve better local tumor control. Our customary approach of using 9–10 Gy/week may not be sufficient treatment for a rapidly proliferating cancer and the use of additional treatments per week would be advisable. A shortening of the overall treatment time to 4 – 4.5 weeks compared to the usual 6 weeks could thus be achieved.

When the measurement of a postoperative CEA level is abnormal, the oncologist must be prepared to do something about it. The finding of an elevated postoperative CEA level may mean embarking on an expensive evaluation for metastatic disease which may be undectable by standard means. Nonstandard approaches for detection of metastatic disease in patients with elevated CEAs in our institution now includes the use on monoclonal anti-CEA antibody scanning. To be eligible for evaluation by the monoclonal antibody technique, the patient must have an elevation in CEA and negative standard radiographs. A variation of the monoclonal antibody technique uses radioimmunoguided surgery where the patient is given the radiolabelled antiCEA antibody and intraoperative exploration is done with a hand-held gamma detector. Metastatic disease may be more successfully detected compared to the surgeon's gross observation and palpation of normal tissues. Unfortunately, neither monoclonal antibody technique using radiographic assessment or immunoguided surgery has resulted in improvement in survival for patients with residual or recurrent disease.

Postoperative XRT treatment has a high probability of controlling microscopic residual pelvic disease with recurrence rates after postoperative XRT ranging between 5% and 20% in a number nonrandomized and randomized trials. In patients with local failure after pelvic XRT, relapse has been described in both the rectum, perirectal soft-tissues and in the pelvic lymph nodes. Our patient presents 2 years after pelvic XRT with a CT scan showing a density in the upper third of the anterior vaginal wall. The clinical exam fails to reveal a palpable mass. The elevated CEA would be consistent with the observation of radiographic evidence of recurrence in a CEA-producing tumor, but otherwise the CEA is not very helpful. The patient needs further diagnostic evaluation to determine the extent of disease.

The utility of serial CEA examinations is unproven (Kievit and Van de Velde 1990). There are some who believe that a biologic predeterminism governs the behavior of metastatic disease which is unaltered by follow-up procedures. According to this view, patients who develop solitary metastatic disease (usually in the liver) will be curable when they become clinically symptomatic of the metastasis. Earlier detection or treatment of metastatic disease in these patients does not affect the outcome, since they are predetermined to have only solitary or limited metastatic disease that can be resected. However, there may be patients with metastatic disease in whom earlier detection can be associated with a greater likelihood of cure. A patient with a small metastasis that has a positive CEA marker, could possibly be detected earlier, and at a stage where the tumor may be more likely resectable. Waiting until the tumor becomes symptomatic could possibly result in the tumor growing large enough where it becomes technically unresectable because of involvement of adjacent organs and structures which preclude surgical extirpation. Another argument for obtaining a follow-up CEA is to detect recurrence earlier in order to decrease the chance of developing a metastasis from a metastasis.

In a patient with elevated CEA, abnormality on pelvic CT scan, and prior history of postoperative pelvic XRT, an evaluation for the extent of metastatic disease would be necessary prior to therapy. If disseminated disease is found, then further local therapy would be futile. However, if metastatic work-up is negative for extra-pelvic disease, a radical approach to treatment with the intent of long-term cure is a reasonable goal. In the patients who have received postoperative pelvic XRT there are limited treatment options. Our philosophy has been to determine resectability and to evaluate the extent of recurrent disease intraoperatively. When a localized perivaginal process is found, wide extirpation with probable removal of the ovaries, fallopian tubes, uterus and a portion of the vagina would be indicated to treat the tumor en bloc. Some patients with central pelvic recurrent adenocarcinoma treated with only surgery may enjoy long-term survival, however most recurrent rectal tumors do not present in this fashion. Most recurrent cancer patients have extensive pelvic disease and it is in these patients where surgical extirpation combined with further radiotherapy can be beneficial. We have seen patients with a similar clinical scenario where the tumor recurrence has infiltrated the previously dissected tissue planes along the posterior and lateral pelvic walls. Recurrent tumor in these locations can compromise the surgical margins because of the close proximity of the bony pelvic walls. Further conventional XRT is limited because most patients have received greater than 45–50 Gy with prior pelvic XRT and we are reluctant to risk the development of severe late XRT-associated morbidity with the use of further XRT. Likewise, we have not used large single fractions of electron beam intraoperative therapy because of the possibility of late radiation morbidity. Instead, we prefer to use an afterloading nylon catheter implant technique to retreat areas of gross or microscopic residual disease. The catheters are placed by the radiotherapist in conjunction with the surgical oncologist in the tumor bed which is defined carefully by the anatomic location of the tumor. Intraoperative tumor biopsies are done with frozen section evaluation during the laparotomy to map out the area for implantation. The catheters are loosely sutured into the tumor site with attention to good parallel geometry and are exteriorized through either an anterior abdominal or perineal wound. After a few days of postoperative recovery the patient is brought to the radiotherapy department for simulation of the afterloading implant. A computer plan is generated and isodose distributions are chosen to radically retreat a small volume adjacent to the resected recurrence. We have employed doses in the range of 50–60 Gy given over 4.5–6 days using low-dose irradiation. A dose rate of 50–70 rads per hour is chosen at a plane of 0.5 cm from the central axis of the implant in the midplane projection. Following the implant, the nylon catheters are removed and the wound heals by primary closure.

In the patient with recurrent, unresectable cancer, tumor size and the infiltrative nature of regrowth generally precludes any further XRT treatment even with extremely tight external fields. In these patients we have used systemic or intra-arterial chemotherapy for palliation (Patt et al. 1985). In view of the possibility of a 10%–20% chance of a tumor regression with systemic chemotherapy, it has sometimes been possible to surgically explore some patients with significant tumor regression. Our experience with recurrent rectal cancer patients presenting after postoperative XRT shows a 40% objective response rate with intra-arterial 5FU and mitomycin. The remission duration, however, is usually short, and the medial survival of this patient population after only chemotherapy treatment is 12 months.

In a patient completing pelvic retreatment by surgical excision plus an afterloading catheter implant to the pelvis, we would consider further systemic "adjuvant" therapy under two conditions. If systemic therapy had not been used previously, its use at this point after giving the patient no evidence of disease (NED) locally would be justifiable. We favor the use of 5FU with modulation by leucovorin or levamisol (or both). In patients who have previously received postoperative adjuvant chemotherapy, no further systemic therapy would be employed.

References

Kievit J, Van de Velde CJH (1990) Utility and cost of carcinoembryonic antigen monitoring in colon cancer follow-up evaluation. Cancer 65: 2580–2587

Krook JE, Moertel CG, Gunderson LL et al. (1991) Effective surgical adjuvant therapy for high-risk rectal carcinoma. N Engl J Med 324: 709–715

Patt YZ, Peters RE, Chuang VP, Wallace S, Fuqua R, Mavglit GM (1985) Palliation of pelvic recurrence of colorectal cancer with intra-arterial 5FU and mitomycin. Cancer 56: 2175–2180

Rich TA (1986) Radiation therapy treatment planning for tumors of the gastrointestinal tract. In: Paliwal BR, Griem ML (eds) A categorical course in radiation therapy treatment planning (syllabus), RSNA Division of Editorial and Publishing Services, Oak Brook, IL, pp 47–55

Rich TA (1992) Chemoradiation for gastrointestinal cancer. Front Radiat Ther Oncol 26: 115–130

Part III Re-irradiation

As to disease, make a habit of two things – to help, or at least to do no harm.

HIPPOCRATES

When the physician is at a loss, it is wiser to do nothing than to recommend what may be injurious.

DAVID CRAIGIE

There is no failure except in no longer trying.

ELBERT HUBBARD

Introduction

Medical and surgical oncologists often fail to understand that if radiation did not benefit the patient the first time, then it is unlikely that irradiation will be effective the second time.

Re-irradiation is often risky if delivered to tubular structures (gut esophagus), brain or spinal cord, or crease areas, such as the groin, axilla or nape of neck. On the other hand, many patients referred for re-irradiation may not live long enough to show tissue damage.

Should undisputable radiosensitivity of a given tumor be evident before re-irradiation is considered? Can the dose given with re-irradiation be lower, or should the dose be at least equal biologically to, or greater than the first time? What are acceptable time intervals between the first and second course? Is hyperthermia worthwhile? Should interstitial implants under general anesthesia be employed? Should re-irradiation be regarded as investigative treatment because of its uncertain scientific basis, or should it be seen as it is standard practice because it is so often done?

In medicine, to convert a failure into a success is a dream of every physician. This rarely happens in oncology. However, every patient's circumstances are unique. Each oncologist commenting upon the following patient histories has a difficult job: to weigh the benefits against the harm of re-irradiation.

20 Recurrent Rectal Carcinoma Post Radiotherapy

R.K. SCHMIDT-ULRICH and N. KAUFMAN

A 66-year-old black man had an abdominal-perineal resection for a poorly differentiated adenocarcinoma of the rectum, stage C2. Hepatic metastases were proven by biopsy. Fourteen months postoperatively, a local pelvic recurrence was given 3000 cGy in ten fractions.

Thirty-six months postoperatively, the pelvic pain has returned. Because of recurrent bladder obstruction, he has to self-catheterize. Computed tomography (CT) shows the presacral mass invading the bladder to be the same size as at the time of irradiation 22 months ago. Liver function tests are abnormal, and the carcinoembryonic antigen (CEA) has climbed from 60 to 130 ng/ml.

1. What are the risks and benefits of re-irradiating this patient's pelvis? How would you do it? Implant?
2. What else would you recommend?
3. What is your experience with neurosurgical procedures for relieving pelvic pain in this situation? Nerve block?
4. [Include other considerations that would influence your recommendation].

Response

Introduction

Patients with symptomatic local recurrences of rectosigmoid carcinoma, with and without metastatic disease, represent one of the most difficult management problems in the oncology practice. Local recurrences represent a component of treatment failure in as many as 92% of the patients and account for a significant number of deaths (RAO et al. 1978; ROMINGER et al. 1985). However, in the majority of patients concomitant metastatic disease tends to be the overriding determinant for patient survival (RAO et al. 1978; ROMINGER et al. 1985). Despite the use of different treatment modalities in patients with recurrent rectosigmoid carcinoma, longer term tumor control can be expected in only a small number of cases (CIATTO and PACINI 1982; DOBROWSKY and SCHMID 1985; WANG and SCHULZ 1962; MAKELA et al. 1989). The unpredictable and vari- able rate of disease progression is the main reason to recommend aggressive management of first postsurgical pelvic recurrences in patients who did not receive the benefit of adjuvant irradiation and/or chemotherapy after surgical resection (FISHER et al. 1988; GUNDERSON et al. 1983; MINSKY et al. 1992). While the overall prognosis of patients with recurrent colorectal carcinoma is poor and unchanged despite the use of irradiation and/or chemotherapy the most optimistic reports, using aggressive management, suggest that as many as 25% of the patients with localized recurrences may experience longer term control of their disease. This short review summarizes the relative effectiveness of palliative treatment methods and weighs the potential benefits and complications of locoregional and systemic treatment approaches.

Re-irradiation

The reported experience with re-irradiation of recurrences of rectosigmoid carcinoma in the pelvis is limited. The majority of these cases when treated after previous high-dose radiotherapy were re-irradiated for recurrent gynecological malignancies, predominantly cervical carcinoma, in patients without evidence of metastatic disease (NORI et al. 1981). In the 56 of 96 patients who had received previous irradiation, high radiation doses during the second treatment course were delivered through permanent implants with or without laparotomy. In about 70% of the patients, symptomatic relief was achieved (NORI et al. 1981). The survival of the patients with recurrent cervical carcinoma was 45%, 20%, and 10% at 1,

Rupert K. Schmidt-Ulrich, MD, Nathan Kaufman, MD, Medical College of Virginia, Department of Radiation Oncology, MCV Station, Box 58, Richmond, VA 23298-0058, USA

2, and 5 years respectively. Severe complications were reported in about 15% of the patients. Another series, reporting on re-irradiation of 40 patients with isolated pelvic recurrences, included ten patients with rectosigmoid carcinomas (PUTHAWALA et al. 1982; SYED 1981). While a second external beam high-dose radiotherapy course was deemed not feasible, temporary implantations were performed using iridium-192, in most patients with recurrent rectosigmoid carcinoma, laparotomy was employed for the construction of these implants (PUTHAWALA et al. 1982). With respect to palliation of pain and bleeding, the success rate was 60%–70%. Of the ten patients, eight experienced local control at the time of death or at a minimum of 2-year follow-up.

Much of the anecdotal experience in the management of recurrent rectosigmoid carcinoma after previous irradiation is not reported in the literature. Implants for after-loading constructed with the help of templates will assure predictable dose distribution and adequate dose delivery for central pelvic recurrences (PUTHAWALA et al. 1982). In addition, these implants do not require laparotomy for placement and can be combined with interstitial hyperthermia (see below). For presacral recurrences, frequent for carcinoma of the rectum, optimal dose delivery with implants alone is more difficult. Here the combined use of implantation with external beam irradiation, using two- or three-field arrangements to the posterior pelvis only, may be more satisfactory. If a significant dose is given with external beam irradiation and the patients can be expected to have a survival longer than 6 months, an accelerated fractionation scheme of twice-daily treatment with fraction sizes around 1.5 Gy should be considered because of selective sparing of late reacting tissues (WITHERS 1985). Boosting to doses beyond 30–40 Gy should always be attempted with a brachytherapy procedure. Implantation techniques for recurrent carcinoma of the rectosigmoid as a means of delivering high-dose irradiation to limited volumes in the pelvis have been described in several reports using intracavitary or interstitial approaches (KAUFMAN et al. 1989; FOURQUET et al. 1985; MINSKY et al. 1990; JACKSON 1980).

Radiation Dose-Response Relationship

Because of the generally poor prognosis of patients with recurrent rectosigmoid carcinomas palliative fractionation schemes with high fraction sizes and low total doses, as used in the case under discussion, will represent inoptimal management in many cases. This position can be supported by a brief review of the dose-response relationships in palliative radiotherapy for rectosigmoid carcinoma.

It has been clearly documented that best use of radiotherapy for advanced stage rectosigmoid carcinomas is the prevention of locoregional recurrences by well-planned, high-dose adjuvant treatment (ROMINGER et al. 1985; GUNDERSON et al. 1983). This may be extended to unresectable primary or recurrent lesions through the use of intraoperative irradiation (GUNDERSON et al. 1983; TEPPER et al. 1986; MINSKY et al. 1991). With respect to recurrent rectal carcinoma, data are less clear because of the generally poor prognosis of these patients. Aggressive approaches including surgical resection have achieved 5-year survival rates as high as 25%, compared with 3% an historical control group at the same institution (WANEBO et al. 1987). These figures compare favorably to results from other experiences (RAO et al. 1978; ROMINGER et al. 1985).

With respect to effective radiation doses for recurrent carcinoma of the rectosigmoid, the literature is confusing because some studies examine symptomatic pain relief as an endpoint, while others measure locoregional tumor control or survival. The first report suggesting a dose-response relationship for advanced rectal carcinoma describes the use of radiation doses in the range of 20–50 Gy where symptoms of pain and bleeding were relieved at lower doses while tumor regression was observed only in the higher dose range (WANG and SCHULZ 1962). Further support for some dose-response relationship is provided by another study showing an 80%–90% relief of the symptoms in patients with inoperable or recurrent colorectal carcinoma (RAO et al. 1978). As a result of different dose/fractionation schedules biological doses in the range of 1000–1700 rets were delivered and resulted in responses of 12%–87%, respectively. These analyses were performed on the entire group of 144 patients only 37 of whom were patients with recurrent inoperable carcinomas. Of the 37 patients irradiated to doses in excess of 50 Gy, five patients, all treated for recurrences of B2 lesions, were alive with follow-up periods of 24–84 months. Of the failing of patients, 86% experienced a local disease failure and 35% died of local disease only. Most impressive dose-response data are available on 113 patients with colorectal carcinoma, 58 with tumor masses measuring more than 5 cm, who were treated with radiation doses ranging from 23–73 Gy using standard fractionation schedules of external beam irradiation (OVERGAARD et al. 1984). Of 77 patients with recurrent disease, only those patients irradiated to more than 56 Gy all showed a response in symptoms with 53% partial and 29% complete response rates. Similarly, the same group of patients experienced a marked benefit in response duration with a complete response at 2 years of 40%, as opposed to less than 10% in patients treated to less than 56 Gy (OVERGAARD et al. 1984).

No dose-response relationship with symptom-free survival could be established in a study of irradiation for recurrent rectosigmoid carcinoma using dose ranges of 35–40 Gy, 41–50 Gy, or more than 50 Gy (PACINI et al. 1986). Symptomatic control was achieved in 80.4% of the patients for about 30% of the patients' life span, irrespective of dose in a patient population that experienced a crude survival of 17.8% at 2 years. In another report, 58 patients were irradiated for presacral pelvic recurrences for rectal carcinomas. Of these, 38 had pain which resolved to varying degrees in 90% (DOBROWSKY and SCHMID 1985). The extent of pain relief was not clearly dependent upon the radiation doses which ranged from 34 to 55 Gy. However, with a mean survival of patients of 19.8 months there was a trend towards improved survival with doses of more than 45 Gy.

Despite some controversy regarding a clear dose-response relationship for recurrent rectosigmoid carcinoma, it is likely that standard fractionation to high doses with careful field planning will have some therapeutic benefit (OVERGAARD et al. 1984). Schedules of extreme hypofractionation, 10 Gy at 4-week intervals to a total dose of 40 Gy plus misonidazole (SPANOS et al. 1987), for advanced pelvic malignancies, about 30% of colorectal origin, resulted in unacceptably high severe late toxicity. These complications were markedly reduced when 14.8 Gy in 4 fractions (3.7 Gy) over 2 days, repeated three times at 4-week intervals were delivered, which yielded 45% response rates (SPANOS et al. 1989).

Studies on local dose escalation using intraoperative electron boosting or implantation in the pelvis included 50 patients with recurrent pelvic rectal carcinoma, 23 of whom received doses in excess of 55 Gy (GUNDERSON et al. 1980). Of the unresectable recurrent rectal carcinomas, all patients failed (three of four in the pelvis) (GUNDERSON et al. 1983).

Hyperthermia

Given the synergistic effect of hyperthermia and irradiation with respect to tumor damage but not normal tissue toxicity (OVERGAARD 1981), there is at least a theoretical advantage of combining the two modalities in the management of rectosigmoid carcinoma recurrent after previous irradiation. With the use of interstitial irradiation, hyperthermia may be useful as an adjunct during that treatment. In a randomized clinical trial, externally applied hyperthermia has only been shown to enhance radiation-induced tumor control with tumors of less than 3 cm diameter (PEREZ et al. 1991). The benefit for larger tumors was compromised by the inability of adequate heating and temperature monitoring (PEREZ et al. 1991). There are currently no data demonstrating that combined hyperthermia and irradiation for recurrent rectal carcinoma in the pelvis will provide a beneficial effect. As many of the pelvic recurrences are discovered at a time when they have reached a significant size, effective heating is unlikely, based on existing clinical experiences (PEREZ et al. 1991; EMAMI et al. 1991).

For recurrent rectal carcinoma in the pelvis, the combined use of intra-arterial chemotherapy and total body hyperthermia to temperatures in excess of 40°C suggest some increased responses in ten patients with a maximum 6 months pain control duration with chemotherapy alone in comparison to 6–18 months of pain control in patients treated with the combination (ESTES et al. 1986).

In a recent report, 71 recurrent or primarily unresectable colorectal tumors were either treated with irradiation plus hyperthermia or with irradiation alone (NISHIMURA et al. 1992) with only ten patients being re-irradiated. The results confirm previous experiences that there may be some improvement in response rates if adequate heating can be achieved that is, tumor temperatures of more than 42°C during three to five treatment sessions can be maintained for more than 20 min. Most severe side effects in the ten patients re-irradiated developed from tumor involvement of the bladder, resulting in bleeding within 6–12 months in patients who had received a cumulative radiation dose of 100 Gy and had persistent tumor (NISHIMURA et al. 1992).

Chemotherapy Alone

A large variety of chemotherapy regimens have been tested (COHEN et al. 1989) in the treatment of recurrent and/or metastatic colorectal carcinoma. To date, 5-fluorouracil (5FU) remains the most commonly used drug for colorectal carcinoma with response rates ranging from 5% to 85% depending on dose levels and its route of administration (COHEN et al. 1989). Overall response rates for 5FU administered through intravenous bolus injections can be expected to be around 20% (COHEN et al. 1989). These and some of the higher reported response rates have to be carefully weighed against severe complication rates as high as 30%. There is evidence that continuous infusion produces higher response rates, measured as tumor regression based on radiographic and imaging studies, with fewer and less severe complications than the delivery of drug by bolus injections (LOKICH et al. 1989). The intra-arterial administration of 5FU in patients with recurrent-rectal carcinoma has produced the highest reported response rates with pain control in 21%–74% of the patients and response durations of several weeks to months (ESTES et al. 1986).

The addition of high- or low-dose folinic acid (FA) (PETRELLI et al. 1989) has improved the tolerance of high-dose 5FU and its therapeutic effect (PETRELLI et al. 1989; ERLICHMAN et al. 1988). In a randomized trial in patients with metastatic colorectal carcinoma escalating doses of 5FU were tested without (control) or with the addition of intermediate or high-dose FA and produced response rates of 12.1%, 18.8%, and 30.3%, respectively (PETRELLI et al. 1989). The significantly increased response rate, measured as 50% reduction in tumor masses, for the 5FU plus high-dose FA group did not translate into any survival advantage. In another randomized trial that compared 5FU and 5FU plus FA, very similar response rates of 7% and 33%, respectively were seen with a significant medial survival advantage for the 5FU plus FA arm of 12.6 months versus 9.6 months for the 5FU group (ERLICHMAN et al. 1988). The response data in this trial were defined as complete or 50% tumor regression 8 weeks after treatment. An even more impressive effect of 5FU on survival is seen if responders are compared to nonresponders (POON et al. 1989).

Relatively impressive results have been reported for the intra-arterial administration of 5FU and mitomycin-C (PATT et al. 1985). Of the 21 patients in the pilot trial, 17 and 15 patients had failed previous radiotherapy and systemic intravenous chemotherapy, respectively. Measurable pain relief by means of reduction in pain medication and subjective pain relief for a mean period of 3.5 months was found in 50% and 75% of the patients, respectively (PATT et al. 1985). Of the patients with elevated CEA levels, 5 of 11 experienced a more than 50% reduction of CEA levels. Dermatitis, neuropathy, and infections occurred at frequencies of 27, 18, and 16% respectively.

Combined Chemo- and Radiotherapy

The concomitant use of high-dose 5FU/mitomycin-C chemotherapy using bolus injections with irradiation has led to unacceptably high complication rates in one experience (WONG et al. 1991). From other experiences it also appears that a continuous course of radiotherapy combined with relatively high doses of 5FU results in significantly increased complication rates (WONG et al. 1991) without a clear benefit in treatment outcome. A randomized trial examining the role of radiotherapy and chemotherapy of 5FU and 1-(2-chloroethyl)-3-(4-methyl cyclohexyl)-1-nitrosourea (MeCCNU) includes 45 patients with unresectable recurrent rectal carcinoma (ROMINGER et al. 1985). Despite radiation doses of more than 50 Gy in most of the patients and the addition of chemotherapy, 95% of the patients failed during the study period with a 26% 2-year survival. The small-bowel complication rate was substantially increased in the combined modality arm. The failure rate in six patients was reduced to 20% and 50%, without and with chemotherapy, respectively, in whom recurrences became resectable after irradiation. Similarly, in a recent pilot study comparing preoperative irradiation without or with 5FU plus FA, the combined modality arm showed superior results with respect to down-staging at the primary and nodal sites and to resectability (MINSKY et al. 1992).

Other Means of Pain Control

Other means of pain control in the pelvis are anesthetic and neurosurgical approaches, as recently reviewed (FOLEY 1985). While temporary or diagnostic nerve blocks can be performed with anesthetics, permanent blocks are achieved by phenol or alcohol infiltration or freezing. The limitations with these techniques are that each nerve subserves sensory function to multiple levels requiring multiple nerves to be blocked for adequate pain control. More extensive epidural or intrathecal blocks with neurolytic agents frequently also cause motor weakness and autonomic dysfunction. Success rates between 22% and 80% of the patients with these procedures have been reported with 1%–13% incidence of significant side effects, such as urinary or rectal incontinence, motor weakness, or parasthesias

(FOLEY 1985). Recent use of continuous anesthetic infusion pumps into the epidural space has achieved good pain control without loss of motor and autonomic function.

As a surgical approach, cordotomy involving the anterior lateral spinothalamic tract in the thoracic spine can be considered. Cordotomy is initially associated with 5% paresis, 20% ataxia, and 10% urinary dysfunction, but carries only a 5% incidence of late complications. Pain relief from cordotomy is 90%, 80%, and 40% immediately 3 months and 5 months post procedure, respectively. Translocation of pain to the contralateral side or another previously unrecognized side can represent limitations in about 15%–20% of the patients.

Conclusions Regarding the Case

Long-term salvage of patients with recurrent rectosigmoid is likely only when surgery and radiotherapy are combined with reported control rates as high as 25%. These control rates may be improved upon by the addition of chemotherapy. Brachytherapy procedures, even in the setting of re-irradiation can be expected to provide effective and lasting palliation in the pelvis in 60%–70% of the patients with reasonable complication rates. Careful consideration has to be given to the relative use of external beam and interstitial/intracavitary irradiation and the use of hyperthermia.

In patients with both recurrent and metastatic rectosigmoid carcinoma who have not had previous chemotherapy, systemic treatment should be seriously considered because of its effectiveness on locoregional palliation in about 20% of the patients, and its potential benefit on survival. The value of initial chemotherapy in patients with local recurrence and distant metastases is that responders may experience a survival advantage and should be considered for locoregional radiotherapy, which is the most effective in providing lasting palliation in the pelvis. Only if these modalities fail should anesthetic and neurosurgical methods of pain control be used.

References

Ciatto S, Pacini P (1982) Radiation therapy of recurrences of carcinoma of the rectum and sigmoid after surgery. Acta Radiol (Oncol) 21: 105–109

Cohen AM, Shank B, Friedman MA (1989) Colorectal Cancer. In: DeVita VT, Hellman S, Rosenberg SA (eds) Cancer: Principles and Practice of Oncology. Lippincott, Philadelphia, pp 946–952

Dobrowsky W, Schmid AP (1985) Radiotherapy of presacral recurrence following radical surgery for rectal carcinoma. Dis Colon Rectum 28: 917–919

Emami B, Myerson RJ, Scott C et al. (1991) Phase I/II Study, combination of radiotherapy and hyperthermia in patients with deep-seated malignant tumors: report of a pilot study by the RTOG. Int J Radiat Oncol Biol Phys 20: 73–79

Erlichman C, Fine S, Wong A, Elhakim T (1988) A randomized trial of fluorouracil and folinic acid in patients with metastatic colorectal carcinoma. J Clin Oncol 6: 469–475

Estes NC, Morphis JG, Hornback NB et al. (1986) Intra-arterial chemotherapy and hyperthermia for pain control in patients with recurrent rectal cancer. Am J Surg 152: 597–601

Fisher B, Wolmark N, Rockette H et al. (1988) Postoperative adjuvant chemotherapy or radiation therapy for rectal cancer: results from NSABP protocol R-01. J Natl Cancer Inst 80: 21–29

Foley KM (1985) The treatment of cancer pain. N Engl J Med 313: 84–95

Fourquet A, Enker WE, Shank B et al. (1985) The value of interstitial radiation in advanced and recurrent colorectal cancer. Endocurie Hypertherm Oncol 1: 113–117

Gunderson LL, Cohen AM, Welch CE (1980) Residual, inoperable or recurrent colorectal cancer. Am J Surg 139: 518–525

Gunderson LL, Cohen AC, Dosoretz DD et al. (1983) Residual, unresectable, or recurrent colorectal cancer: external beam irradiation and intraoperative electron beam boost and resection. Int J Radiat Oncol Biol Phys 9: 1597–1606

Jackson BR (1980) Iridium implants in treatment of anorectal carcinoma. Dis Colon Rectum 23: 145–150

Kaufman N, Nori D, Shank B et al. (1989) Remote afterloading intraluminal brachytherapy in the treatment of rectal, rectosigmoid, and anal cancer: a feasibility study. Int J Radiat Oncol Biol Phys 17: 663–668

Lokich JJ, Ahlgren JD, Gullo JJ, Philips JA, Fryer JG (1989) A prospective randomized comparison of continuous infusion fluorouracil with a conventional bolus schedule in metastatic colorectal carcinoma: a mid-atlantic oncology program study. J Clin Oncol 7: 425–432

Makela J, Haukipuro K, Laitinen S et al. (1989) Surgical treatment of recurrent colorectal cancer. Arch Surg 124: 1029–1032

Minsky B, Shank B, Nori D et al. (1990) Subtotal resection and intraoperative brachytherapy in recurrent rectosigmoid and rectal cancer. Endocurie Hypertherm Oncol 6: 31–40

Minsky BD, Cohen AM, Enker WE et al. (1991) Radiation therapy for unresectable rectal cancer. Int J Radiat Oncol Biol Phys 21: 1283–1289

Minsky BD, Cohen AM, Kemeny N et al. (1992) Enhancement of radiation-induced down-staging of rectal cancer by fluorouracil and high-dose leucovorin chemotherapy. J Clin Oncol 10: 79–84

Nishimura Y, Hiraoka M, Akuta K et al. (1992) Hyperthermia combined with radiation therapy for primarily unresectable and recurrent colorectal cancer. Int J Radiat Oncol Biol Phys 23: 759–768

Nori D, Hilaris BS, Kim HS et al. (1981) Interstitial irradiation in recurrent gynecological cancer. Int J Radiat Oncol Biol Phys 7: 1513–1517

Overgaard J (1981) Fractionated radiation and hyperthermia: experimental and clinical studies. Cancer 48: 1116–1123

Overgaard M, Overgaard J, Sell A (1984) Dose-response relationship for radiation therapy of recurrent, residual, and

primarily inoperable colorectal cancer. Radiother Oncol 1: 217–225
Pacini P, Cionini L, Pertoli L et al. (1986) Symptomatic recurrences of carcinoma of the rectum and sigmoid. Dis Colon Rectum 29: 865–868
Patt YZ, Peters RE, Chuang BP et al. (1985) Palliation of pelvic recurrence of colorectal cancer with intra-arterial 5FU and mitomycin. Cancer 56: 2175–2180
Perez CA, Pajak T, Emami B et al. (1991) Randomized Phase III study comparing irradiation and hyperthermia with irradiation alone in superficial measurable tumors: final report by the RTOG. Am J Clin Oncol 14: 133–141
Petrelli N, Douglass HO, Herrera L et al. (1989) The modulation of fluorouracil with leucovorin in metastatic colorectal carcinoma: a prospective randomized phase III trial. J Clin Oncol 7: 1419–1426
Poon MA, OConnell MJ, Moertel CG et al. (1989) Biochemical modulation of fluorouracil: evidence of significant improvement of survival and quality of life in patients with advanced colorectal carcinoma. J Clin Oncol 7: 1407–1418
Puthawala AA, Syed AM, Fleming PA et al. (1982) Re-irradiation with interstitial implant for recurrent pelvic malignancies. Cancer 50: 2810–2814
Rao AR, Kagan AR, Chan PY et al. (1978) Effectiveness of local radiotherapy in colorectal carcinoma. Cancer 42: 1082–1086
Rominger CJ, Gelber RD, Gunderson LL et al. (1985) Radiation therapy alone or in combination with chemotherapy in the treatment of residual or inoperable carcinoma of the rectum and rectosigmoid or pelvic recurrence following colorectal surgery. Am J Clin Oncol 8: 118–127
Spanos WJ, Wasserman T, Meoz R et al. (1987) Palliation of advanced pelvic malignant disease with large fraction pelvic radiation and misonidazole: final report of RTOG Phase I/II study. Int J Radiat Oncol Biol Phys 13: 1479–1482
Spanos WS, Guse C, Perez C et al. (1989) Phase II Study of multiple daily fractionations in the palliation of advanced pelvic malignancies: preliminary report of RTOG 8502. Int J Radiat Oncol Biol Phys 17: 659–651
Syed AM (1981) Interstitial irradiation as a salvage technique. Int J Radiat Oncol Biol Phys 7: 1613–1614
Tepper JE, Cohen AM, Wood WC et al. (1986) Intraoperative electron beam radiotherapy in the treatment of unresectable rectal cancer. Arch Surg 121: 421–423
Wanebo HJ, Gaker DL, Whitehall R et al. (1987) Pelvic recurrence of rectal cancer. Ann Surg 205: 482–495
Wang CC, Schulz MD (1962) The role of radiation therapy in the management of carcinoma of the sigmoid, rectosigmoid, and rectum. Radiology 79: 105
Withers HR (1985) Biologic basis for altered fractionation schemes. Cancer 55: 2086–2095
Wong CS, Cummings BJ, Keane TJ et al. (1991) Combined radiation therapy, mitomycin-C, and 5FU for locally recurrent rectal carcinoma: results of a pilot study. Int J Radiat Oncol Biol Phys 21: 1291–1296

21 Breast Cancer Re-irradiation

R.D. PEZNER

In 1985, a 64-year-old woman had an excisional biopsy, axillary dissection and irradiation to the breast, supraclavicular and internal mammary regions for a stage II adenocarcinoma of the left breast. Post irradiation, she was placed on tamoxifen. Two years postoperatively she noticed lymphedema of her left arm. A biopsy of enlarged nodes in the supraclavicular region revealed adenocarcinoma compatible with the primary in the left breast.

1. Under what general circumstances do you re-irradiate locoregionally in breast cancer?
2. Under what circumstances would you re-irradiate this woman's supraclavicular axillary region?
3. Are there any pitfalls in re-irradiation here?
4. [Include other considerations that would influence your recommendation].

Response

Numerous retrospective studies and several prospective randomized trials have demonstrated that postmastectomy radiation therapy (RT) for the chest wall and regional lymph node sites is highly effective in reducing the risk of breast cancer recurrence at these sites. Several retrospective studies have also demonstrated that radiation therapy is of significant palliative benefit for locoregional recurrence of breast cancer. Symptoms are frequently relieved, long-term locoregional tumor control can be achieved in many patients and, in some cases, long-term disease-free survival can result. In comparison, patients who develop tumor recurrence in previously irradiated locoregional sites are usually not good candidates for RT. The sum of two courses of RT to regional lymph node sites such as the supraclavicular fossa (SCF) would carry a high risk of possible radiation injury to skin, subcutaneous tissue, clavicle, brachial plexus and/or lymphatic and venous channels. The risk of such debilitating radiation therapy complications as brachial plexopathy, arm lymphedema, skin ulceration and osteoradionecrosis of the clavicle would exclude most patients from consideration of further RT. Moreover, the reason that a repeat course of RT is being entertained is because tumor recurred in spite of a previous course of RT. Such a tumor might inherently be more resistant to radiation than most breast cancers, possibly due to cellular DNA repair mechanisms. This point would lead to the conclusion that repeat RT to a site of in-field recurrence is not likely to produce as much benefit as even the first course which failed to control the tumor. Still, there are infrequent circumstances where a repeat RT course is appropriate to recommend. In order to make this determination, a comprehensive evaluation is necessary.

The patient must first be evaluated for extent of disease. The patient's history should especially emphasize symptoms which might be suspicious for brachial plexopathy, arm lymphedema, paralysis of a recurrent laryngeal nerve and skeletal pain. The physical examination should specifically search for these abnormalities. In addition, the physical examination should also search for metastatic disease to the opposite breast, contralateral lymph nodes and hematogenous metastatic sites. Diagnostic tests should be performed to search for hematogenous metastases. If a patient has distant metastases, it may not be in her interest to take the risks of a repeat course of RT if that treatment cannot encompass all known sites of disease. The evaluation should therefore include chest radiograph, nucleotide bone scan and computed tomography (CT) scan of the liver and adrenal scans. A CT chest scan might also be performed since it would be superior to a plain chest radiograph in searching for metastatic disease in the internal mammary nodes, mediastinal nodes, lungs and pleural surfaces. Suspicious findings on history, physical examination or diagnostic scans may need further evaluation to determine if other sites of metastatic disease are present.

Richard D. Pezner, MD, Division of Radiation Oncology, City of Hope National Medical Center, 1500 E. Duarte Road, Duarte, CA 91010–0269, USA

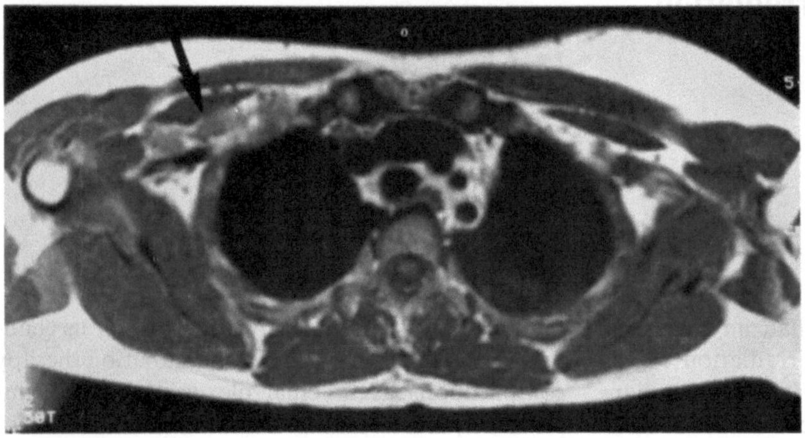

Fig. 1. Magnetic resonance imaging (MRI) scan of 32 year old woman with supraclavicular recurrence of breast cancer one year following modified radical mastectomy. While physical examination showed a 3.5 cm. right supraclavicular lymph node without axillary adenopathy, MRI scan showed an 8 × 3 cm. chain of lymph nodes located deeper along the course of the subclavian vein (*arrow*)

The extent of regional tumor recurrence needs to be determined as accurately as possible. The case example describes concurrent onset of arm lymphedema at the time of discovery of SCF node recurrence. This raises the possibility of tumor present deep in the soft tissues of the high axilla and base of the neck, too deep to be palpated on physical examination. Even if the patient did not have findings such as arm lymphedema or brachial plexopathy, a small SCF lymph node recurrence may be just the "tip of the iceberg." Frequently, much bulkier disease is found in the soft tissues deep to the palpable node (Fig. 1). The disease may represent a "geographic miss" of the previous RT course which may have limited the SCF tumor dose to a depth of perhaps 3 cm deep to the anterior skin surface. A CT scan of the neck and high axilla will frequently demonstrate bulky tumor in this region. Personal experience, however, suggests that magnetic resonance imaging (MRI) may be more sensitive than CT scanning for this part of the body. Disease missed by CT scan is frequently evident on MRI scan. Extent of disease can be determined in the three projection planes provided by MRI scanning. Biopsy of the suspicious lymph node (as already performed in this case) should be performed to confirm that malignancy is the basis for recommending RT to a previously irradiated site.

Last, but not least, the records of the previous RT course must be reviewed in detail. Estimated total doses should be determined for critical structures such as the anterior skin surface, clavicle, brachial plexus and spinal cord. Total doses to regions of current tumor involvement should also be determined.

In assessing whether or not to recommend a course of RT, it should be recognized that in most cases of SCF node recurrence in a previously irradiated site, a repeat RT course will not be indicated. In some cases, distant metastases will be discovered, leading to a recommendation for systemic chemotherapy or hormonal manipulation. In other cases, there will be no evidence of disease outside of the supraclavicular region but the previous RT course precludes the possibility of delivering even a palliative dose without high risk of complications. If the previous RT course and the proposed palliative course involve fraction sizes of 180–200 cGy per day, there would be a high risk of complications if the sum of both courses delivered more than 4600 cGy to the spinal cord and/or 6500 cGy to the brachial plexus.

RT may be recommended in the following situations:

1. The total radiation dose to the brachial plexus and lymphatics from the previous treatment course was modest. This may be the case if a low energy electron beam was employed for most of or all of the first course of treatment of the supraclavicular fossa. In this circumstance, the limiting critical structures would be the anterior skin surface and the clavicle.
2. The disease volume is small, that is, the SCF recurrence is small and MRI scan shows no other evidence of tumor as a basis for the arm lymphedema. In this circumstance, it is assumed that lymphedema is a complication of previous cancer treatment and/or infection in the hand or arm.
3. Tumor recurrence is producing such disabling symptoms that palliative RT is recommended even if there is evidence of distant metastases, massive tumor in the SCF region or previous high-dose RT. Pain from local tumor growth, bone invasion or malignant brachial plexopathy would

be the principal indication under this category. Arm lymphedema by itself would not be an indication for palliative RT since the dose from the second course in addition to the dose from the initial treatment would sum to a total lymphatic dose which would put the patient at high risk of treatment-induced lymphedema. Thus the patient would be trading lymphedema due to cancer for lymphedema due to RT.

We can make the following treatment recommendations:

1. Small SCF lymph node recurrences may be treated by small RT fields. If the previous treatment course involved a photon beam, the repeat course should be delivered by an electron beam of appropriate energy such that the 80% depth isodose line encompasses the deepest extent of tumor. Concurrent external hyperthermia by either microwaves or ultrasound may increase the chances of local control. The SCF, however, is often a difficult site for optimal hyperthermia delivery. Microwaves may not penetrate to a sufficient tissue depth to adequately heat the deepest extent of tumor. Ultrasound may not be able to heat tumor behind the clavicle. A recommended dose schedule might be 3000 cGy in ten fractions, five fractions per week. An alternative dose schedule is 3200 cGy in eight fractions, two fractions per week.
2. Larger tumors in regions with modest previous RT doses to the brachial plexus and lymphatics may be treated with modest palliative radiation doses to relieve pain or reduce tumor volume. Anterior and posterior opposed equally weighted photon beam fields are recommended to avoid high daily doses to any part of the irradiated volume. A dose of 4000–5000 cGy at 180–200 cGy per fraction might be recommended with the patient's understanding and informed consent that there would be risk of complications involving skin, clavicle and brachial plexus. In this circumstance, spinal cord tolerance should not be exceeded. Ultra-sound hyperthermia may be recommended in those cases where it is able to deliver adequate heating of the entire tumor volume.
3. For expedient palliation of tumor-induced pain in a patient with bulky tumor and/or widespread metastases, a dose schedule of 2500–3000 cGy, 180–200 cGy per fraction, five fractions per week, frequently provides gratifying, although transient, pain relief.

22 Cauda Equina Syndrome Secondary to Lymphoma

W.T. Moss

One year ago, this 59-year-old woman developed rapidly progressive leg weakness. An exploratory laparotomy and biopsy of a large retroperitoneal mass demonstrated a diffuse large cell lymphoma. A partial response with cyclophosphamide, Adriamycin (doxorubicin), Oncovin (vincristine)-bleomycin (CHOP-BLEO) and subsequent delivery of 3600 cGy to the whole abdomen still did not make the mass disappear on computed tomography (CT), so cytoxan and prednisone were added. The mass began to grow and this was accompanied by nausea, vomiting, neutropenia, fever, and leg weakness.

A bone scan was positive at T6–8 and L3–4. Magnetic resonance imaging (MRI) showed a pathologic fracture of L4, associated with a left psoas mass and soft tissue infiltration of the epidural space. The hemoglobin level was 9.5 g/l.

1. Would you re-irradiate this patient? What limits this option?
2. What would you guess her life expectancy to be.
3. If the previous ports included the lower thoracic spine, would you re-irradiate the spinal cord?
4. What are the chances that re-irradiation will enable this patient to walk?
5. [Include other considerations that would influence your recommendation]

Response

This patient has an incurable, poorly responsive, progressive, symptom-producing diffuse histiocytic lymphoma. The gastrointestinal (GI) symptoms, fever, and recurrence of her leg weakness are ominous findings and warrant a relatively short life expectancy.

William T. Moss, MD, Oregon Health Sciences University, Division of Radiation Oncology, 3181 S.W. Sam Jackson Park Road, Portland, OR 97201, USA

Therapeutic Options to Be Considered

Other than withholding treatment, what are the therapeutic options to be considered for this patient who has developed what is ordinarily considered an oncologic emergency?

Re-irradiation of this patient's spinal cord is associated with an increased risk of cord damage which should be avoided if a reasonable alternative is available. Two attempts with good chemotherapy have failed. Meaningful response from further chemotherapy is highly unlikely. The neurosurgeon will certainly not recommend cord decompression in a patient with this advanced disease and limited longevity.

Thus, there are problems with each of three options ordinarily considered for patients with spinal cord compression by lymphoma. Of the three, re-irradiation has the greatest promise. The likelihood of early response is good and the likelihood that radiation-induced cord damage will appear during her short life is slim. Furthermore, the alternative to re-irradiation is progressive cord compression with all of its sequelae.

When is it ethically appropriate to subject a patient who has only a few months to live to a short course of radiation therapy which has an excellent chance of preventing lower extremity paralysis and fecal and urinary incontinence? There is no single "correct" answer to this question. This is certainly not the time or place for a highly zealous radiation oncologist. However, if this patient is judged to have several months longevity, emergency irradiation is indicated.

The patient should be informed compassionately and deliberately that irradiation will greatly diminish the chances that she will become paralyzed and incontinent for the remainder of her life. The risks of treatment and of no treatment must be spelled out. Most patients will elect irradiation if it is not too demanding of their immediate physical strength.

Technical Considerations

The aspects of this patient's lymphoma with which we are concerned is described as a "large, soft tissue psoas mass with infiltration of the epidural space and involvement of vertebrae L3–4." T6–8 are involved as shown by bone scan. The fact that this patient has obvious lymphoma at one cord level should not blind us to the possibility that other levels of the cord may be involved. Review of the physical examination and MRI should, so far as is practical, exclude this possibility. The volume of epidural space infiltration plus a generous superior and inferior margin (4–6 cm at least) and right and left margins (2–3 cm lateral to the vertebrae) are sufficient. There is no need to encompass the entire "large" psoas mass or vertebrae T6–8.

A previous dose of 3600 cGy has been given to the infradiaphragmatic segment of the spinal cord. (This is presumed to have been given at a daily fraction of 2.0 Gy or less since it was given as a part of whole abdominal irradiation.) An initial dose of 3.0 Gy per daily fraction would be redu-ced after two to three fractions to 2.5 Gy per daily fraction and carried to a total cord dose of 2850 cGy in about 11 fractions. In addition, dexamethasone (96 mg/day) should be started as soon as diagnosis is made, continue for 3–4 days, then tapered over 2 weeks.

Benefits and Risks

A large proportion (perhaps 80%) of patients with progressive leg weakness from cord or nerve root compression who have not already developed permanent vascular occlusion will improve with steroids. A rapid response to steroids is a good indicator that there will likely be a good response to irradiation. In any case, this cell type, early diagnosis of compression and immediate administration of steroids and irradiation promise an excellent response in the large majority of patients. The dose recommended is sufficient to prevent recurrence during her short life.

The only risk from this treatment, assuming her blood counts, etc., are able to tolerate the irradiation, is in the unpredictability of radiation-induced cord damage when the spinal cord is re-irradiated. The frequency of radiation myelitis and the timing of this myelitis after re-irradiation are unpredictable with our current knowledge. However, when the uncertainties associated with re-irradiation of spinal cord compression are matched with the certainties associated with no further treatment, it has not been difficult for us to make the decision to irradiate a second time. Finally, if we were certain this patient had only 2 weeks to live, we would withhold irradiation. If we felt she might live 2 months or more we would likely recommend irradiation.

Part IV Recurrence

The National Cancer Institute and the American Cancer Society spend next to nothing on noncurative cancer treatment. They are interested in prevention; they are interested in curative treatment, surgery or chemotherapy. But they spend very little money on pain control or psychosocial issues.
One reason for the neglect of palliative care is this country's dedication to a high-tech pursuit of a cure, even though most leading cancer primaries – of the breast, colon, stomach, pancreas, and lung – remain incurable once they have spread.

DECLAN WALSH

Los Angeles Times, August 27, 1991

Introduction

At no point is the radiation oncologist's judgement more crucial than at the appearance of recurrent cancer. These frequently unsolvable clinical problems are often disguised by our mentors as "challenges." Dr Porter Storey (Hospice, Texas Medical Center) said: "You know, it's just easier for an oncologist to say 'Come back and see me next month' when he knows the patient will be bed-bound and too weak to be able to, instead of saying 'Gosh, you're getting really weak. We know your cancer is progressing. How about we get you into a hospice service because you are going to die from this soon.' That's a tough message."

About 5% of recurrences appear as a solitary metastasis, with a previous long disease-free interval. Should these be treated with abbreviated treatment regimens? Should metastatic foci from cancer of the thyroid or some cancers of the kidney be treated differently because of their longer survival histories?

Biopsy of a suspected recurrence may be contraindicated when the site is close to a vital structure (e.g., the aorta). Should the oncologist be satisfied with a fine needle aspirate result which reads as "compatible with metastatic carcinoma?"

Should our consultative recommendations on patients with recurrences from cancer of the rectum be similar, whether the recurrence is $5 \times 5 \times 5$ cm or $15 \times 15 \times 15$ cm? Hope for palliation is not tantamount to actual accomplishment.

The discussants in the following case histories have had to consider many patient variables, though many factors, some stated, but most unstated, check memories of their own experiences, including both their failures and successes, and finally recommend a clinically effective approach for a noncurable patient.

23 Chest Wall Recurrence Post Breast Cancer Surgery

P.W. Edland

One year ago, this 54-year-old woman had an inflammatory adenocarcinoma of the right breast. She was treated with doxorubicin (Adriamycin) plus surgery, but a lesion recurred on the chest wall in 2 months. A complete response with cyclophosphamide, methotrexate, and 5-fluorouracil (CMF) was then observed.

1. Would you now irradiate the left chest wall or simply follow the patient? Why?
2. Does inflammatory adenocarcinoma of the breast merit surgery as primary treatment?
3. What is the place of irradiation?
4. [Include other considerations that would influence your recommendations].

Response

In my opinion, if 1 year has elapsed since the original treatment and there is no evidence of systemic disease on careful workup (to include blood chemistry and bone scan), I would recommend irradiation of the chest wall and probably would include the regional lymphatics. Since the patient has survived 1 year, the chances for a durable maintenance of disease-free survival is enhanced, although the fact that a lesion recurred on the chest wall may indicate that seeding distantly – which is not yet apparent – has already occurred. I believe that the quality of life for this patient will be enhanced, since the patient is at high-risk for developing another chest wall recurrence, probably in the range of 30%, in view of the original presentation, despite original treatment with Adriamycin and later with CMF following recurrence on the chest wall.

I would prefer integration of radiotherapy (Shaefer et al. 1987; Fields et al. 1989; Moore et al. 1991) in tandem to neoadjuvant chemotherapy and surgery if the patient's breast lesion is operable, on a preplanned basis, since locoregional recurrence is so very high despite chemotherapy and mastectomy in inflammatory breast cancer. I do not feel that surgery up front should be utilized, but if there is a good response to chemotherapy and the lesion becomes operable, then I would favor this treatment followed by radiotherapy to the chest wall and regional lymphatics, rather than simple observation after mastectomy. Surgery should not be utilized as the initial tool in inflammatory cancer, and I do believe neoadjuvant chemotherapy should be utilized. If the lesion does not become resectable, then breast radiotherapy may be utilized and surgery may follow, depending upon the response to radiotherapy.

The usual place of irradiation, in my opinion, is to treat lesions which after chemotherapy remain unresectable per primum, or to prevent locoregional recurrence in patients who undergo neoadjuvant chemotherapy and surgery for what is, in effect, locally advanced breast cancer presenting in an inflammatory state. Surgery may well seed the tumor, and the intradermal lymphatics are usually involved by tumor, so that I do not believe that initial surgery should be employed in inflammatory carcinoma of the breast, which is essentially a clinically diagnosed entity.

This patient would have been better served by the use of neoadjuvant chemotherapy (in this case Adriamycin was employed) followed by surgery, if the lesion was operable, but then followed by postoperative radiotherapy and further integrated chemotherapy (if indicated). The amount of postmastectomy chemotherapy would depend upon the number of cycles given preoperatively. There has been improvement in the disease-free survival of inflammatory breast cancer by utilizing this technique and cycling of modalities. Radiotherapy is utilized to improve quality of life and prevent local recurrence, which can be very distressing to the patient, usually given as a postmastectomy form of integrated therapy. The biggest problem continues to be distant spread of cancer. Of course,

Robert W. Edland, MD, Department of Radiation Oncology, Gundersen Clinic, 1836 South Avenue, La Crosse, WI 54601, USA

locoregional radiotherapy will not affect distant disease if it has already occurred. At 1 year, however, I believe the patient is in a different biological situation than on initial presentation. For this reason, since it was not utilized in integrated fashion following mastectomy, I would suggest it be employed at this point, since the patient may still have a significant survival interval, having survived the first year after treatment without evidence of distant disease.

References

Fields J, Kuske R, Perez C, Fineberg B, Bartlett N (1989) Prognostic factors in inflammatory breast cancer. Cancer 63: 1225–1232

Moore M, Ihde J, Crowe J, Hakes T, Kinne D (1991) Inflammatory breast cancer. Arch Surg 126: 304–306

Shaefer P, Alberto P, Forni M, Obradovic D, Pipard G, Krauer F (1987) Surgery as part of a combined modality approach for inflammatory breast cancer. Cancer 59: 1063–1067

24 Aggressive Abdominal Lymphoma

M.J. Miller

A 76-year-old man presented with lower gastrointestinal (GI) bleeding. The cause was a diffuse non-Burkitt's lymphoma of the terminal ileum which had perforated. While a resection was performed, disease remained around the right ureter and invaded the small bowel and mesentery. He had lost 20 lbs. Two months after the completion of six courses of cyclophosphamide, hydroxydaunomycin (doxorubicin), Oncovin (vincristine) (CHOP), a very large (12 × 12 × 6 cm) right lower quadrant subcutaneous mass was biopsied and diffuse non-Burkitt's lymphoma was diagnosed. The mass grew during treatment with etoposide (VP-16) and prednisone.

1. What would your goal be in irradiating this mass? What is your treatment volume: the mass, the whole pelvis, or the whole abdomen?
2. What dose would you give? What are the possible complications?
3. What can irradiation be expected to achieve in a patient who recurs 2 months after CHOP?
4. [Include other considerations that would influence your recommendation].

Response

The treatment of choice for primary small-bowel lymphoma, which often is of a high-grade histology, involves some form of resection followed by combination chemotherapy with or without irradiation. If the tumor mass is resectable, an enbloc resection is potentially curative. A study by Taggert et al. (1986) reported a 48% 5-year survival after resection versus a 12% 5-year survival following an incomplete surgical resection.

Selected factors of poor prognosis in small-bowel lymphoma are extremes of age, large size of primary, extraregional lymph node involvement, bone marrow involvement and incomplete surgical resection, all of which are present in the above patient.

While 30%–50% of patients with diffuse aggressive lymphomas may be cured with combination chemotherapy such as CHOP, prednisone, doxorubicin, cyclophosphamide, etoposide, cytarabine, bleomycin, oncovin, methotrexate, leucovorin (ProMACE–CytaBOM), methotrexate, bleomycin, adriamycin, cyclophosphamide, oncovin, leucovorin (M-BACOD), and methotrexate, leucovorin, doxorubicin, cyclophosphamide, vincristine, bleomycin, prednisone, co-trimoxazole, ketoconazole (MACOP-B), those patients who fail induction therapy or relapse shortly after achieving a complete remission (CR) have a grave prognosis. Conventional salvage regimens provide only a 0%–10% chance of significant disease-free survival. Other approaches such as autologous bone marrow transplantation (ABMT), although promising, are still investigational and certainly not indicated for most situations, especially in the elderly patient.

In the above patient, there is little to offer in the way of effective therapy to significantly increase survival without undue morbidity. The role of irradiation in this patient is limited. With the knowledge of bowel perforation, invasion of small-bowel mesentery and the large size of the known mass, any radiation portal short of total abdominal or near total abdominal would be grossly inadequate to have an effect on the course of this patient's disease. It is always enticing when dealing with a radiosensitive tumor such as a lymphoma to give a "little bit" of radiation, but when large volumes are required over the abdomen in an elderly patient with previous surgery and heavily treated with chemotherapy, the therapeutic ratio is narrow and any dose used will result in bowel and bone marrow toxicity.

Whether this patient should receive further palliative chemotherapy depends on his general medical condition, his social support systems, and his ability for self care, which allows him to maintain a feeling

Michael J. Miller, MD, Department of Radiation Oncology, Southern California Permanente Medical Group, 4950 Sunset Boulevard, Los Angeles, CA 90027, USA

of well-being, despite his illness. Problems with nausea, vomiting, diarrhea, anorexia, and fatigue, all of which can occur as a result of abdominal irradiation, will adversely affect this patient's quality of life and possibly even decrease survival. Before further therapy is offered, these issues should be discussed with the patient and his family, and I would recommend supportive care and pain management when needed.

References

Taggert DP, McLatchie G, Durie CW (1986) Survival of surgical patients with carcinoma, lymphoma, and carcinoid of the small bowel. Br J Surg 73: 826–828

25 Retroperitoneal Recurrence from Anal Canal Carcinoma

S.O. Asbell

Five years ago, a 53-year-old woman was treated for squamous cell carcinoma of the anal canal with metastasis to the right inguinal lymph nodes with 5-fluorouracil (5FU)/mitomycin concurrently with 3000 cGy.

Presently she is complaining of severe progressive back pain, with a computed tomography (CT) scan showing a mass destroying lumbar vertebrae starting in the psoas and extending to the iliac region, with an associated hydronephrosis. Left supraclavicular lymphadenopathy was accompanied by a negative chest radiograph.

1. How would you manage this patient? With irradiation? With chemotherapy?
2. How would you discuss the risks of antineoplastics versus the benefits?
3. When would you refer to hospice?
4. How does the disease-free interval influence your treatment recommendations?
5. [Include other considerations that would influence your recommendation].

Response

A 53-year-old woman was treated for squamous cell carcinoma of the anal canal with metastasis to the right inguinal lymph nodes with 5FU/mitomycin and concurrently with 3000 cGy. She presents with progressive back pain and a CT scan showing a mass destroying the lumbar vertebrae starting in the psoas and extending to the iliac region with an associated hydronephrosis. Incidentally, there was a left supraclavicular lymph node, although the chest X-ray was negative. This patient presented with advanced stage disease, her tumor having spread to the retroperitoneum and left supraclavicular fossa. She is unlikely to be a candidate for chemotherapy alone because of the progressive pain and the destruction of the vertebral body.

For this reason, my recommendation would be a combination of therapy again, a course for palliation consisting of local radiation to the lumbar vertebrae and chemotherapy with 5FU/mitomycin. If the supraclavicular fossa lymphadenopathy does not regress on chemotherapy alone, subsequent radiation to this area would also be administered. No less than 4000 cGy should be delivered despite the chemotherapy because of the bony destruction. She could be managed with radiation alone if refusing chemotherapy, however, there is probably subclinical metastasis in the lung or liver unbeknownst to us by current means of evaluation and chemotherapy might prevent these from becoming clinically symptomatic.

We are dealing with palliation. It would not be inappropriate to treat only for local pain to the lumbar retroperitoneal adenopathy, however, in all likelihood the supraclavicular node would progress and cause neurologic dysfunction some time in the future from brachial plexopathy so that if it was not treated by chemotherapy and then followed, local radiation could also be administered, probably from a single anterior approach. The abdomen, however, should be treated from an anterior-posterior approach to at least 4000 cGy.

It would be a shame to refer this patient to hospice because the disease would progress until her death and her pain would continue. The disease could be controlled with narcotics, but it could become disabling and to the point that she would not be able to walk when the epidural space has been invaded, and this would leave her paraplegic for the rest of her life. As this may not be a rapidly growing tumor, considering that she had lived with progression of disease for the 5 years since she underwent low-dose radiation with chemotherapy, an equal or longer interval may occur before her death.

My decisions would be as follows: a 53-year-old woman could serve a useful time as a family member and mother were she able to live another 5 years.

Sucha O. Asbell, MD, Albert Einstein Medical Center, Department of Radiation Oncology, 5501 Old York Road, Philadelphia, PA 19141–3096, USA

Referring her to hospice would diminish that opportunity since she could have a better quality of survival outside it, although at this point I doubt that she is curable. I would be aggressive also because of the probability of continued expansion of the tumor into the epidural space and the probability of causing cauda equina syndrome, loss of bowel and bladder function, and paraplegia. Her pain could probably be controlled. She may get some regression of metastasis that are small in nature and therefore remain asymptomatic from any subclinical disease. Placing her in a hospice would just allow her to go for a relatively long period without treatment and probably develop increasing pain, poor control, poor walking and a bad quality of survival. The fact that she lived 5 years free of clinical evidence of disease also speaks for the slow growth of the tumor and consideration for aggressive palliation.

26 Pelvic Pain

B.S. ARON

The patient is a 61-year-old black man who presented with stage IV adenocarcinoma of the prostate. For 2 years he was in remission on lupron and flutamide. However, for the recent 3 months he has had progressive back, right hip and right leg pain. Bone scan showed new lesions in the right sacroiliac and lumbar-thoracic spine regions.

1. Do you need any other studies before irradiation?
   a. X-rays? Why?
   b. Magnetic resonance imaging (MRI)? Why?
   c. Computed tomography (CT)? Why?
2. Any blood tests indicated?
3. Do you need a bone biopsy?
4. What dose fraction would you recommend?
   a. Hemibody?
   b. Local fields?
   c. Include all vertebrae?
5. [Include other considerations that would influence your recommendation].

Response

Diagnosis

Prostate adenocarcinoma, stage IV, with bone metastasis.

Plan of Therapy

Palliation of pain from bone metastasis.

Evaluation of Patient

1. Parameters of pain – length of time, location, severity (drug dosage to relieve pain), mobility of patient, performance status.
2. Parameters of prostate cancer – physical examination, prostate-specific antigen (PSA), complete blood count (CBC), liver and bone chemistries (especially change with time), chest X-ray, plain X-rays of areas of abnormal bone scan, serum testosterone (to see if adequate androgen ablation has been achieved), evidence of extraosseous metastases – peripheral lymph nodes, liver, lymphangitic or nodular lung metastases, etc. If evaluation showed inadequate androgen ablation, I would suggest orchiectomy. If plain X-rays appeared "normal" in the presence of an abnormal bone scan, would then evaluate further with MRI scan. If PSA is increasing and there are sclerotic bone lesions diagnostic of prostate cancer, we would proceed to treatment as follows:
3. If the metastases are limited to bone and the patient is in good general condition, not anemic, and his pain not severe (managed by codeine, etc.) and if the patient is ambulatory, I would consider using 198-rhenium, 89-strontium, or some other isotope and delay local radiation therapy.
4. If the patient's condition is similar to that described above, but the pain is severe and prevents ambulation, thereby necessitating morphine-type drugs, I would consider administering local radiation therapy to painful areas. Local radiation would be given to the lumbar spine and sacroiliac joint areas with in an inverted "T"-shaped field, including, if necessary, lower thoracic vertebral bodies as parallel opposed ports (POP) fields to midline dose of 30 Gy per ten fractions of 300 cGy on linear accelerator of 4–10 MV (ARCANGELI et al. 1989).
5. If the patient's condition were poor, i.e., anemia, significant weight loss, confined to bed, and the pain was severe, I would consider administering same volume of irradiation but would deliver the treatment in a shorter period of time, as 20 Gy/5 treatments of 400 cGy (TONG et al. 1982; BLITZER 1985).
6. If there is evidence of liver or lung metastases (especially lymphangitic lung) cytotoxic

Bernard S. Aron, MD, University of Cincinnati Medical Center, Department of Radiation Oncology, Cincinnati, OH 45267–0757, USA

chemotherapy would be given if patient could tolerate chemotherapy – radiation given if no response or if adequate chemotherapy could not be tolerated by patient. Dosage would be as in C above/or could be 10 Gy (VARGHA et al. 1969) per single treatment (limit area 150 cm^2). The parameters to be followed to evaluate response would include subjective pain relief, narcotic dosage, and perhaps the change in PSA level (in patients with limited bone metastasis).

Hemibody radiation (600 cGy/single dose upper or 800 cGy/single dose lower hemibody with steroids, etc) would be considered for diffuse disease, as in B above, for patients whose lesions could not be easily encompassed by local fields. High-dose radiation (4000 cGy/3–4 weeks) would be considered for patients with solitary or few weight-bearing, predominantly lytic lesions, so as to facilitate healing (recalcification) of these lesions (MATSUBAYASHI et al. 1981).

References

Arcangeli G, Micheli A, Arcangeli G, Giannovelle D, LaPasta O, Tollis A, Vitullo A, Ghira S, Benassi M (1989) The responsiveness of bone metastases to radiotherapy – the effect of site, histology, and radiation dose on pain relief. Radiother Oncol 14: 95–101

Blitzer P (1985) Re-analyses of the RTOG Study of the palliation of symptomatic osseous metastases. Cancer 55: 1468–1472

Matsubayashi T, Koga H, Nishiyama Y, Tominaga S, Sawada T (1981) The reparative process of metastatic bone lesions after radiotherapy. Jpn J Clin Oncol 11: 253–264

Tong D, Gelleck L, Hendrickson F (1982) The palliation of symptomatic osseous metastases. Cancer 50: 893–899

Vargha Z, Glicksman A, Boland J (1969) Single-dose radiation therapy in the palliation of metastatic disease. Radiology 93: 1181–1184

27 Lumbar Pain Post Nephrectomy

C.M. Chahbazian

For 5 years, an 84-year-old woman had been followed for a large left renal mass which had slowly increased in size until it was removed for symptoms of gross hematuria and left flank pain. Diagnosis was adenocarcinoma of the kidney. Eight months postoperatively she complained of right lumbar pain. Computed tomography (CT) showed a large right paralumbar mass invading the vertebrae. She was disoriented as to place and her illness.

1. Would you request a biopsy of the paraspinal mass?
2. What time-dose relationship would you use?
3. To what extent do you modify management based on age?
4. Would an earlier nephrectomy have prevented the metastasis?
5. [Include other considerations that would influence your recommendation].

Response

I would not request a biopsy of the paraspinal mass in view of the fact that the picture described above falls well into the pattern of metastasis from the carcinoma of the kidney, and since it would be relatively difficult to biopsy this area, especially in an 84-year-old person. Under these circumstances, the development of a paraspinal mass and the destruction of adjoining vertebrae would be strong presumptive evidence of metastasis that would justify consideration of palliative therapy.

For the time-dose relationship, I would use 300 cGy in ten fractions to a total of 3000 cGy, at the level of the tumor mass described above. I would not modify management bases on age in this particular case since the main purpose is palliation of pain and, if this could be done in a relatively short period of time, it would be well-justified in an 84-year-old woman, as well as in someone 20 years of age.

An earlier nephrectomy could theoretically have prevented the metastasis mentioned above, although carcinomas of the kidney generally metastasize rather readily, but I would have to go by the general principle of early diagnosis and early treatment as the best approach in the management of any type of malignancy.

The special considerations in this case would include treating only the bulk of the metastasis and adjoining destroyed vertebrae, primarily to relieve pain, but in this process the whole volume of the tumor may not be included in the field of treatment if a good part of the only remaining right kidney will come into the field of treatment. Therefore, I would take every precaution of avoiding treating most of the only remaining right kidney, even if it is harboring some residual tumor. Most likely, in this particular case, the pain is related to the destroyed vertebra and the bulk of the tumor rather than the entire process of metastasis.

Chahin M. Chahbazian, MD, Radiation Oncology Medical Group of Southern California, Anaheim, CA 92807, USA

28 Bone Metastases Post Breast Cancer

C.M. Chahbazian

A 52-year-old woman who had cancer of the right breast, stage II, was treated 3 years previously with a modified right radical mastectomy followed by adjuvant chemotherapy. She did well for about 2.5 years, but about 6 months ago she presented with moderate pain in the left hip area, radiating to the left lower extremity. X-rays indicated lytic changes of the left iliac bone at the left sacroiliac region, confirmed also with increased uptake on bone scan, as well as many different other areas of increased uptake in the skeletal system. In view of the high degree of suspicion of metastasis, the patient began palliative chemotherapy since then and has repeated numerous regimens without relief of pain. Her general condition has deteriorated rapidly over the past 6 months, and the pain has become increasingly worse. She has at the present time been referred for consideration of palliative radiation to the left sacroiliac region. It should be noted that her general condition remained markedly deteriorated at this time.

1. Should the patient have been treated with radiation therapy 6 months ago?
2. How long should one wait after chemotherapy before beginning palliative radiation therapy?
3. What would be the time:dose relationship?
4. What could be expected from the course of radiation therapy?

Response

Chemotherapy could be administered for a short while, but if no relief of pain followed within a matter of a few weeks to 2 months, then consideration should be given to local radiation therapy earlier.

The time:dose relationship would be either 300 cGy in ten fractions to a total dose of 3000 cGy through anteroposterior/posteroanterior (AP:PA) fields, or 500 cGy in four fractions to a total dose of 2000 cGy to the same area can be considered. With radiation therapy, good pain palliation would be obtained within a relatively short period of time, i.e., 2–4 weeks.

General Considerations

Most adequate palliation could be offered to patients with metastatic carcinoma of the breast, especially to the skeletal system with a prompt and short course of radiation therapy. It is true that in this particular case, the patient had diffuse skeletal metastasis, so systemic therapy would have been justified, but only for a short period of time. If she had responded well to chemotherapy, then radiation therapy could have been withheld; however, in view of the fact that she had continued with moderate to severe pain, waiting with additional courses of chemotherapy had not served the purpose well, and in fact by the time the patient came for radiation therapy, her general condition had deteriorated markedly. This makes the administration of radiation therapy, even for palliative intent on a more adequate and reasonable basis, difficult. The plea in these cases is to not delay the start of palliative radiation therapy if patients are not showing good response to chemotherapy.

Chahin M. Chahbazian, MD, Radiation Oncology Medical Group of Southern California, Anaheim, CA 92807, USA

29 Leukemic Meningitis

M. Tomé

A 7-year-old white boy was treated for a diagnosis of acute lymphoblastic leukemia 3 years ago. Part of his treatment included 40 mg methotrexate intrathecally and 1800 cGy brain irradiation. Presently he has relapsed with symptomatic leukemic meningitis. His bone marrow remains negative.

1. What are the treatment goals – palliative or curative?
2. Does he need systemic therapy?
3. What is the recommended technique of irradiation?
4. Is this patient a candidate for bone marrow transplantation (BMT)? If so, what is brain tolerance to "chemo radiation?"
5. What should the parents be told about the patient's intellectual level after radiation? Growth after craniospinal irradiation?
6. [Include other consideration that would influence your recommendation].

Response

In the practice of pediatric oncology, leukemia is by far the most common malignancy in children. Acute lymphoblastic leukemia (ALL) accounts for approximately 80% of childhood leukemia (Halperin et al. 1989). The child that has been described in this clinical case, fortunately, is an uncommon situation that is seen in today's practice. With the development of successful chemotherapy for the treatment of ALL, the central nervous system (CNS) became the most common site of relapse. Approximately 33%–60% of patients develop CNS recurrence if they did not receive adequate prophylaxis (Kun and Pinkel 1977). Introduction of CNS prophylaxis either with chemotherapy alone, radiotherapy alone, or a combination of the two has decreased the rate of CNS recurrence, but unfortunately it is not zero. Approximately 10% of children will relapse in the CNS after adequate prophylaxis.

CNS recurrence is a dismal sign. The control of these patients in the long run is very poor. The literature states that approximately only 20% of these patients are long-term survivors (Kun et al. 1984). Although survival is low, I would be aggressive with this patient and treat him for cure since he relapsed when off therapy. CNS relapse, even without bone marrow relapse needs aggressive treatment. Once there is CNS relapse, there is systemic failure. I would recommend treating the child with systemic and intrathecal chemotherapy to reinduce the child, and then this would be followed by cranial-spinal radiotherapy.

The technique of cranial-spinal radiotherapy has become fairly standardized. Most often the cranial field plus a separate spinal field with megavoltage beams are used. Sometimes two separate spinal fields have to be used depending upon the height of the child. Treatments are given 5 days per week, treating each field once per day. The patient is best treated with opposed beams with dose calculated to midplane. The spinal fields are treated with posterior ports. It is very important to account for the junction, so that an overlap is avoided. Cranial-spinal irradiation should be reserved for children with overt CNS leukemia at time of diagnosis or patients who develop CNS relapse. The standard dose would be 2400 cGy in 12 fractions to the cranium, with 1200 cGy to the spinal axis. This should all be done after his cerebrospinal fluid (CSF) has been cleared with intrathecal chemotherapy. If the patient has a positive leukemic infiltration of the brain on magnetic resonance imaging (MRI) or computed tomography (CT) scan, then I would recommend a higher dose to the cranium. The dose to the cranium would be increased to approximately 3000 cGy.

Regarding BMT, if this child had an human leukocyte antigen (HLA)-matched donor, then I would consider him for allogenic BMT once he was in remission, since the outcome of salvage

Michael Tomé, MD, Department of Radiation Oncology, Southern California Permanente Medical Group, 4950 Sunset Boulevard, Los Angeles, CA 90027, USA

chemotherapy and craniospinal radiotherapy is less than 20%. I would not have offered him cranial-spinal radiotherapy if the induction regimen of his BMT included total body irradiation. If he was to be transplanted after cranial-spinal radiotherapy then I would recommend chemotherapy only as induction prior to BMT, since the probability of developing CNS complications after prophylactic radiation, cranial-spinal radiotherapy, and total body irradiation would be extremely high, on the order of 100%.

Complications from cranial or cranial-spinal irradiation for prophylaxis are well-documented but the complications of cranial-spinal radiotherapy with CNS recurrence are difficult to document since the salvage rate of these patients is so poor. When spinal axis radiation is used, if the dose is maintained to below 2000 cGy, then I would not be concerned with bone hypoplasia. Areas of concern are: (1) neurotoxicity, (2) neuroendocrine abnormalities, and (3) secondary malignancies. BLEYER (1981), found that therapy-induced encephalopathy increased as the number of treatment modalities increased. Leukoencephalopathy can occur after doses of 2400 cGy with chemotherapy. In one study, severe encephalopathy developed post treatment in nine of the 20 children who received 2400 cGy to the cranium followed by intravenous methotrexate at a dose of more than 40 mg/m^2 per week (BLEYER et al. 1973). Methotrexate appears most neurotoxic when given during or after radiation therapy. There has been one retrospective study which looked at 107 patients treated for CNS recurrence (OCHS et al. 1985). The aim of the study was to look for neurotoxicity. Patients were treated with different modalities. The initial problem was that many patients received different combinations of chemotherapy, three different methods of CNS prophylaxis, and not all patients received the same treatment modalities for CNS relapse. All patients received intrathecal methotrexate plus at least 2400 cGy for CNS prophylaxis or as part of their therapeutic regimen for their CNS relapse. Patients who were cured received a second course of radiotherapy consisting of an additional 2400 cGy. Serious neurotoxicity was found in 79 patients who eventually died of leukemia or infection. Twenty-eight patients were survivors, nine patients had seizures associated with intrathecal methotrexate, seven had episodes of status epilepticus, and five have recurrent seizures while receiving anticonvulsant therapy. Intelligence quotient (IQ) evaluation was performed in this population. One year post CNS relapse, a mean IQ of 83 ± 16 (range 67–110) was found.

In conclusion, although we would anticipate measurable reduction in learning abilities after such an aggressive treatment, it is difficult to say if the neurotoxicity is secondary to the treatment alone or the combination of treatment and the disease. We will need to further analyze these children to determine the long-term side effects of chemoradiotherapy in children with CNS relapse.

References

Bleyer WA (1981) Neurologic sequelae of methotrexate and ionizing radiation: a new classification. Cancer Treat Rep 65

Bleyer WA, Dicke JC, Chabner BA (1973) Neurotoxicity and elevated cerebrospinal methotrexate concentration in meningeal leukemia. N Engl J Med 289: 770–773

Halperin EC, Kun L, Constine LS, Tarbell NJ (1989) Pediatric radiation oncology. Raven, New York (Chap. 2)

Jenkin RDT (1979) Radiation in the treatment of meningeal leukemia. Am J Pediatr Hematol Oncol 1: 49–58

Kun L, Pinkel D (1977) Meningeal leukemia: control vs cure. Int J Radiat Oncol Biol Phys 2: 371–373

Kun L, Camitta B, Mulhern R et al. (1984) Treatment of meningeal relapse in childhood lymphoblastic leukemia: international results of craniospinal irradiation. J Clin Oncol 2: 359–364

Ochs J, Rivera G, Aur RJ et al. (1985) Central nervous system morbidity following an initial isolated central nervous system relapse and its subsequent therapy in childhood acute lymphoblastic leukemia. J Clin Oncol 3: 622–626

30 Extensive Recurrence of Colon Carcinoma

D.H. Hussey

A 61-year-old man had a B2 adenocarcinoma of the sigmoid colon resected 2 years ago. He fainted, and on admission he was found to have a hemoglobin level of 5 g/dl. Colonoscopy showed a recurrent lesion at 12 cm. Computed tomography (CT) scan showed hydronephrosis of bilateral pelvic kidneys. Liver metastases, ascites and bilateral pleural effusions were also present. His creatinine level was 4.2 mg/dl.

1. What is your experience with irradiation of postoperative, recurrent pelvic colonic masses?
2. Would a colostomy be enough?
3. If the kidneys were in normal position, would that alter your recommendation?
4. [Include other considerations that would influence your recommendation].

Response

This patient is clearly not curable, and consequently the goal for any subsequent treatment would be palliation. Palliative treatment may be used to relieve actual symptoms or impending symptoms. Treatment to relieve impending symptoms has been termed "pre-emptive palliation." In this case, the symptoms that might require palliation include (1) gastrointestinal hemorrhage, (2) impending bowel obstruction due to recurrent tumor at the anastomotic site, and (3) renal failure due to hydronephrosis. There is also a possibility that the patient will subsequently develop pain due to invasion of the lumbosacral nerves, or direct extension to bone.

There are a number of other factors that can influence the decision to deliver or not deliver palliative treatment. These include the extent of the disease elsewhere in the body, the patient's general life expectancy, the likelihood of relieving the symptoms in a timely manner with doses that can be tolerated, the duration of the proposed course of treatment, and the risk of normal tissue injury. In general, more aggressive treatment is used in patients whose disease is progressing slower and in patients who have a longer life expectancy, than in those who will die of their disease within the next several weeks.

Another factor that should be kept in mind is the mode of death. Death from renal failure or hepatic failure is usually relatively painless and trouble-free for the patient, whereas death associated with nerve impingement, bony metastasis, pulmonary dysfunction, or massive exsanguination can be difficult for the patient and his/her family.

Based on the facts given, I would not use radiation therapy in the palliative management of this patient. I reached this decision because the patient has multiple liver metastases, ascites, and bilateral pleural effusion, which indicate that his disease is rapidly progressing. He is not likely to live long enough to receive significant palliation from irradiation even if it were able to be given. Besides, the symptoms requiring palliation in this case can be managed by other means. His impending colonic obstruction could be well-palliated with a colostomy, and his renal failure would probably respond to ureteral stenting.

One uncertainty with the case as stated is the cause of the patient's anemia. It is very likely that the anemia is at least partly due to intestinal hemorrhage, although his renal failure could be a contributing factor. Certainly, his anemia should be corrected. Transfusions can be a problem in patients with renal failure. Because of this, his ureters should probably be stented to improve his renal function prior to transfusion. If stenting is not possible, a percutaneous nephrostomy should be considered, although this could be problematic because the patient has bilateral pelvic kidneys.

An added problem in this particular case is that the patient has bilateral pelvic kidneys. Consequently, palliative radiation therapy would be difficult to deliver even if it were indicated for other reasons. However, even if the kidneys were in normal position in this patient, I would not advocate palliative

David H. Hussey, MD, Department of Radiation Oncology, University of Iowa College of Medicine, 200 Hawkins Dr., # W 1892 GH, Iowa City, IA 52242-1009, USA

radiation. This is because the patient already has liver metastases, ascites, and bilateral pleural effusion and can be managed by other means.

This tumor might not have recurred had the patient received postoperative radiation therapy following his low anterior resection 2 years previously. Adjuvant pelvic radiation has been shown to decrease the incidence of local recurrence from 35%–50% with surgery alone to 10%–20% with surgery and postoperative radiation therapy in stage B2–3 and stage C rectal carcinoma patients (Hoskins et al. 1985; Romsdahl and Withers 1978; Tepper et al. 1984). Unfortunately, because of the pelvic kidneys, elective irradiation would not have been feasible.

References

Hoskins B, Gunderson LL, Dosoretz D et al. (1985) Adjuvant postoperative radiotherapy in carcinoma of the rectum and rectosigmoid. Cancer 55: 61–71

Romsdahl M, Withers HR (1978) Radiotherapy combined with curative surgery. Arch Surg 113: 446–453

Tepper JE, Gunderson LL, Orlow E et al. (1984) Complications of intraoperative radiation therapy. Int J Radiat Oncol Biol Phys 10: 1831–1839

31 Local Recurrence from Cancer of the Rectum

W.A. Bethune

At age 49, a white woman had a right tubo-ovarian abscess removed. Nine months later a 10 cm rectal mass was found at the level of the uterine fundus. An extended abdominal-perineal resection (APR) revealed a moderately differentiated adenocarcinoma of the rectum invading the right ovary and uterine myometrium. Two months post APR, a necrotic lesion which was associated with a 7 cm pelvic mass was diagnosed as adenocarcinoma on biopsy in the vaginal vault. Liver function tests (LFTs) were normal, but the carcinoembryonic antigen (CEA) level was 24.5 ng/ml.

1. Is there a "best" means of palliation available?
2. Can the latest pelvic mass be sterilized? How?
3. How radiosensitive are large rectal masses, or their extensions or recurrences?
4. [Include other considerations that would influence your recommendation].

Response

In this situation, as in most areas of medical practice, a systematic approach is necessary prior to a treatment decision, focusing on the medical history and physical findings initially and followed by appropriate investigations.

The first question is whether the pelvic pathology is symptomatic. Is there pain or bleeding? Is there swelling of the extremities, are there urinary symptoms such as frequency, urgency or hematuria. In the past medical history one needs to know if there is a history of any other abdominal surgery. Perhaps there is a history of multiple surgeries. These questions, of course, bear on the risk of complications if high dose external beam radiation is administered.

The systemic enquiry should address whether there are any symptoms of metastatic disease, e.g., headache, cough, or bone pain. The physical examination should assess first of all the patient's general condition. Is the patient in a good nutritional state? Is the patient ambulatory? Is the patient fully active and able to work? The physical examination should assess also for signs of metastatic disease. Is there any adenopathy? Is the liver enlarged? Are there signs of a pleural effusion? Are there areas of bone tenderness? Is there any evidence of neurological deficit? (In my experience cerebellar involvement is particularly common with rectal cancer). The examination of the pelvis should confirm the size of the pelvic disease. Is there one contiguous mass? Is it mobile or is it fixed to the pelvic sidewall or other structures?

Having completed the history and physical examination, attention should be turned to special investigations. The investigations should include complete blood count (CBC), chemistry panel, and urinalysis. Radiological studies should include a chest radiograph and computed tomography (CT) of the abdomen and pelvis.

Having completed the above assessment, a treatment decision can be contemplated. Assuming that no disease is found outside the pelvis, the initial crucial decision with respect to locally recurrent rectal cancer is whether or not the mass can be resected surgically. For a patient this young, an aggressive approach would, in general, be warranted.

In a personal review of 38 patients developing recurrent disease in the pelvis in Saskatchewan, four of 14 resected and radiated patients survived 5 years, and none of 24 patients treated with radiation alone survived 5 years (Bethune 1987). Although this difference mainly reflects selection bias, the trend is clear. Similar results were obtained in other studies (Pearlman et al. 1987). Approximately 10% of patients treated by radiation alone survive 5 years (Ciatto and Pacini 1982; Dobrowsky and Schmid 1985; Overgaard et al. 1984; Rominger et al. 1985). If resection is to be attempted and an intraoperative radiation suite is available, the exploration should preferably be carried out in such a facility. There have been encouraging anecdotal reports of the use

Wyman A. Bethune, MD, Stony Brook University Hospital, Department of Radiation Oncology, Stony Brook, NY 11794–7028, USA

of intraoperative therapy for locally recurrent rectal cancer (COHEN et al. 1980).

Depending on the findings at surgery, an intraoperative boost of 1500–2000 cGy may be administered, either to gross tumor, if the lesion is unresectable, or to the tumor bed, if it is resectable. In any case, surgical clips should be placed at sites of residual tumor or in the tumor bed and surgical exploration should include careful inspection and palpation of the mesentery and liver.

Having completed surgical exploration, if appropriate, we are now faced with either a patient who has had all disease completely resected and is potentially a long-term survivor, or one who has unresectable disease and whose treatment has to be considered palliative. In general, unresected rectal cancer of this size cannot be sterilized by radiation treatment. Both the curative and the palliative situation require external beam radiation. Even an asymptomatic patient with an unresectable mass should be treated, as the likelihood of early development of symptoms is great. This is so called prophylactic palliation, and I would favor this type if pre-emptive intervention in this situation for prevention of symptoms such as pain and bleeding.

For the patient with resectable disease the treatment recommended would encompass the whole pelvis initially with a four-field box technique. A total of 4500 cGy should be administered to this volume in 25 fractions of 180 cGy. Following this, a smaller volume tailored to the CT abnormalities should be taken to a dose of 1000 cGy in five fractions again with a four-field box technique or a three field technique with wedges where appropriate. Thus the total dose is 5500 cGy in 6 weeks.

For the patient with unresectable disease external beam radiation treatment is also indicated. The fractionation pattern offered depends on the general condition of the patient. If the patient is active with a good performance status a more protracted course of treatment can be administered. As for patients with unresectable disease, an initial dose of 4500 cGy should be administered in 25 fractions of 180 cGy by a four-field box technique. Subsequently a boosting dose of 1600 cGy in eight fractions should be administered by a four-field or three-field technique. This high total dose gives the patient the best chance of prolonged freedom from local progression while maintaining a reasonable balance between the risks of treatment and its potential benefits.

For patients with poor performance status or patients with metastatic disease, one must strike a balance between the need to deliver a dose high enough to shrink the tumor and prevent local symptoms and the need to not unduly prolong the course of treatment in a dying patient. In this situation, pelvic radiation with a four-field technique is again recommended, but the dose would be fractionated differently to 3500–4000 cGy in 14–16 fractions of 250 cGy each. Most patients will tolerate 3500 cGy with 250 fractions and, depending on clinical response, some patients can be taken to 4000 cGy.

In addition to the general approach described above, a few additional points should be mentioned.

Preoperative Radiation

If this patient had been found to have locally unresectable tumor initially, a planned re-evaluation after 4500 cGy was given would have been appropriate. At that point, an assessment of operability might show conversion from a locally unresectable situation to a resectable situation. At this point, following a 4-week rest period, surgical resection would be carried out. Again, with a patient this young aggressive intervention is warranted.

Chemotherapy

The mainstay of chemotherapeutic treatment for rectal cancer is the use of 5-fluorouracil (5FU). This agent produces objective responses in approximately 20% of treated patients. More recently 5FU has been combined with leucovorin, and the combination is said to produce responses in as high as 40% of treated patients. In either case, the duration of response is brief, being only 2–4 months at best. For the patient we are discussing here, chemotherapy has no role as an isolated modality. The role of chemotherapy as a radiation sensitizer has been reported in a study of the use of 5FU and mitomycin combined with radiation for patients such as this one (WONG et al. 1991). The combination was highly toxic and did not increase the number of long-term survivors over radiation alone. This was also the result of an earlier study of radiation plus 5FU and 1-(2-chloroethyl)-3-(4-methyl cyclohexyl)-1-nitrosourea (methyl-CCNU) (ROMINGER et al. 1985).

Extent of Surgery

For a patient this young, the possibility of anterior exenteration to remove the recurrent tumor has to be considered. This extent of surgery may be necessary to remove all tumor. This must be fully discussed with the patient prior to surgery. She must understand that surgical removal of all tumor by exenteration might give her a better chance of survival but at the cost of a decrease in quality of life, from the necessary additional ostomy. The patient must make the decision about this prior to exploration.

Intraoperative Brachytherapy

In a few clinics in the United States, a patient such as this would be considered for the insertion of radioactive isotopes to residual tumor placed during the surgical exploration. Permanent implants of iodine-125 or removable implants of iridium-192 may be employed. I am not in favor of this practice as it is never possible to do a good implant in this setting and the contribution to local control is negligible. This practice drives up the patient's hospital bill and may increase surgical complications. The cost-benefit and risk-benefit ratios of this approach are, in my view, unfavorable.

Quality of Life and Cost

As alluded to earlier, a major consideration with respect to the extent of surgery, and to a lesser extent the use of chemotherapy in combination with radiation, is treatment toxicity and quality of life. The patient must participate in management decisions affecting her quality of life.

It is a sad fact that most of the money spent on an individual patient's health care is spent during the last 3 months of life. Cost containment needs to be a more urgent objective of patient management than it is at present. The current system of provider reimbursement does little to foster the will for containment. Management alternatives should be decided with this factor in mind, moreso than is the current practice nationally.

Apart from prescribing and administering radiation to the patient she will need the support of her physicians, nurses, and social workers in coping with her emotional needs. She must understand that she will always be able to get help if she needs it, with such matters as pain control, etc. Although recurrence is a very serious problem much can done to help these patients.

References

Bethune WA (1987) Carcinoma of the rectum: 508 patients with failure analysis and implication for adjuvant therapy. J Can Assoc Radiol 38: 206–216

Ciatto S, Pacini P (1982) Radiation therapy of recurrences of carcinoma of the rectum and sigmoid after surgery. Acta Radiol 21: 105–109

Cohen AM, Gunderson LL, Wood WC (1980) Intraoperative electron beam radiation therapy boost in the treatment of recurrent rectal cancer. Dis Colon Rectum 23(7): 453–455

Dobrowsky W, Schmid AP (1985) Radiotherapy of presacral recurrence following radical surgery for rectal carcinoma. Dis Colon Rectum 28: 917–919

Overgaard M, Overgaard J, Sell A (1984) Dose-response relationship for radiation of recurrent, residual, and primarily inoperable colorectal cancer. Radiother Oncol 1: 217–225

Pearlman NW, Donohue RE, Steigmann GV, Ahnen DJ, Sedlacek SM, Braun TJ (1987) Pelvic and sacropelvic exenteration for locally advanced or recurrent onorectal cancer. Arch Surg 122(5): 537–541

Rominger CJ, Gunderson LL, Gelber ED, Conner N (1985) Radiation therapy alone or in combination with chemotherapy in the treatment of residual or inoperable carcinoma of the rectum and rectosigmoid or pelvic recurrence following colorectal surgery. Am J Clin Oncol 8(2): 118–127

Wong CS, Cummings MB, Keane TJ, Dobrowsky W, O'Sullivan B, Catton CN (1991) Combined radiation therapy, mitomycin-C, and 5FU for locally recurrent rectal carcinoma: results of a pilot study. Int J Radiat Oncol Biol Phys 21(5): 1291–1296

Part V Miscellaneous

There are circumstances in which the split between scientific and practical medicine is so great that the learned physician can do nothing, while the practical physician knows nothing. Lord Bacon has said 'sciencia est potentia' (science is authority). Knowledge which is unable to support action is not genuine – and how unsure is activity without understanding! This split between science and practice is rather new; our century and our country has brought it into being.

RUDOLF VIRCHOW

Introduction

Since there is neither a clinical staging system nor a classification of metastases based on dysfunction (the KARNOFSKY status being too vague for most organ systems), "Miscellaneous" might be the title of this entire volume. It is a fact that although the majority of patients irradiated are incurable, there is more written on the management of mycosis fungoides than pain, palliation, or advanced locoregional cancer. Today irradiating a patient without a histologic diagnosis is common, but it was even more common before the advent of aspiration cytology and stereotaxic-guided biopsies. Yet there are virtually no articles on treating without a histologic diagnosis. Recently, I saw a gadolinium-enhanced magnetic resonance imaging (MRI) scan of the brain. There was a lesion in the corpus collosum and one in the parietofrontal region on the same side. A neuroradiologist interpreted the study as showing a single rather than two separate lesions, because both lesions shared a common edematous region. The majority of radiation oncologists favored biopsy even though all agreed the probability of the abnormality being glioblastoma multiforme was 95%. This scenario, with perhaps a different consensus because of different images and a different history, occurs weekly in our practice. Although this scenario, in our practice, occurs most often with cerebral lesions, the same controversy occurs with bone, liver or pulmonary (suspected) metastases without a tissue diagnosis.

Should a painful bone be irradiated if the patient has a history of cancer when the etiology is unclear? When should a suspected solitary metastasis be biopsied? When a patient has signs of epidural cord compression in the face of normal cerebrospinal fluid and imaging studies, should irradiation be delivered on the basis of the neurological examination?

High-tech and statistics have changed the clinical nature of our specialty. Firstly, high-tech now shares the oncologist's environment. Imagine, the patient's tumor site can be outlined by the diagnostic radiologist on computed tomography (CT) or MRI, the dosimetrist and the planning technologist can together structure a 90% isodose curve to cover the tumor volume defined by the diagnostic radiologist. The work of the dosimetrist and the planning technologist can be checked by the physicist. The radiation oncologist can wait in his office for the port film.

Secondly, statistics have liberated us from clinical judgement. No more anecdotal case reports, just "what is the *p* value." And what a house of mirrors forms the infrastructure of modern statistics, the positive slogan on most randomized studies being "outcome has been improved 15% by treatment X," when only 24 patients of the 400 entered have survived. But all the high-tech and statistics cannot remove clinical judgement from evaluating the patient with incurable cancer. Neither statistics nor computers can think, are flexible, or have common sense and humility, the latter two most needed for assessing these patients with advanced cancer.

Enough chatter; let us read what the discussants have to say.

Part V Miscellaneous

Introduction

32 Pelvic Pain

R.R. DOBELBOWER, J.A. BATTLE, and S. GUPTA

A 74-year-old white man had a total colectomy for well-differentiated adenocarcinoma of the rectum (B2) at 7 cm associated with many adenomatous and villoadenomatous polyps and a cecal carcinoma in situ and metastases to the liver. Due to the liver metastases, the operative procedure omitted the perineal portion and left a anorectal stump (Hartman pouch) in the pelvis. The patient was placed on chemotherapy for 1 year. Three years later, he began complaining of pelvic pain which over the next 6 months became refractive to an infusion of morphine sulfate. A biopsy of the anorectal remnant 6 months previously, at the onset of pelvic pain, showed no tumor, but now there was a tender rectal mass which was a new palpatory finding and on computed tomography (CT) was seen to invade the distal sacrum.

1. Should this patient have received radiation to the pelvis initially?
2. Will the pain be relieved by radiation now? For how long? Dose-time volume?
3. If the distal rectal margin was positive for adenocarcinoma, would your recommendations have been different?
4. Any comments regarding pain medicines, hospice, nerve block, etc?
5. [Include other considerations that would influence your recommendation].

Response

We are presented with a 74-year-old man who was treated with total colectomy because of a Stage B2 well-differentiated adenocarcinoma of the rectum at 7 cm from the anus. Presumably, the total colectomy was performed because of the many adenomatous and villadenomatous polyps. We trust that the in situ carcinoma was discovered in the cecum incidentally. Because of hepatic metastases, perineal resection of the anorectal stump was not performed. The current problem is one of progressive pelvic pain, which has become refractory to morphine sulfate infusion. Although a biopsy of the anorectal remnant 6 months previously was negative, there now is a tender rectal mass which has been found to invade the distal sacrum. This almost certainly represents a recurrent adenocarcinoma and, in the face of the physical findings and the CT scan evidence of sacral invasion, we would not insist on a biopsy prior to institution of palliative treatment.

We wonder why radiation therapy was not applied to the pelvis postoperatively. Consideration was obviously given to adjuvant treatment, as the patient did receive chemotherapy (agent unspecified) for 1 year. In view of the hepatic metastases, this was probably appropriate. However, the incidence of local recurrence is stage B2 rectal cancer (24%–43% after "curative" resection) is high enough to warrant local radiation therapy. The fact that the anorectal stump was left in place increases the chance of local recurrence to well above 50%. With modern radiation therapy techniques (multiple custom-shaped fields; high energy, deeply penetrating beams; techniques to image and displace bowel from the pelvis during treatment, etc) the morbidity of adjuvant pelvic irradiation in such a situation is really quite low.

The question for us now is: "what to do?" We have an elderly man with refractory pelvic pain, undoubtedly due to recurrent rectal cancer invading the sacrum. How aggressive should one be in this situation? Is simple pain management treatment enough? Should a trial of radiation therapy be undertaken? Unfortunately we do not have a great deal of information regarding the current status of the disease, much less the patient. Had the time interval between operation and the recurrence of cancer been much shorter (the patient has been rather lucky to survive 3.5 years!) the answers to the above questions might be much easier. Now we are faced with a cancer that

Ralph R. Dobelbower, MD, PhD, FACR, J.A. Battle, MD, S. Gupta, MD, Medical College of Ohio, P.O. Box 10008, Toledo, OH 43699–00088, USA

is apparently behaving in an indolent manner and, with no further information, we might expect him to live many months or perhaps even a year or so. Clearly, if this is the case, aggressive palliative efforts are not contraindicated. On the other hand, if we have information that would seem to indicate a relatively rapid demise (brain metastases, extensive metastases in liver or lung), we would certainly think that high-risk aggressive palliative efforts would not be appropriate.

In general, we are opposed to expending expensive medical resources in situations where there is little to be gained; however, in the current case, we should consider obtaining a chest X-ray as well as liver function studies and (if indicated by neurologic examination) a CT scan of the brain. At this juncture, we wish to point out that a careful history and physical examination by the radiation oncologist is probably of greater importance than any imaging study to assess whether or not the patient is a candidate for any palliative treatment and to determine the aggressiveness of that treatment. If we are able to convince ourselves that this patient has a reasonably long life expectancy (in excess of 1 year) then we personally would recommend a very aggressive approach to the recurrent rectal lesion: preoperative radiochemotherapy followed by resection of the pelvic mass and partial sacrectomy with intraoperative electron beam therapy (IOEBRT) to the sacral stump and the tumor bed. In our experience we have found that this combination of modalities is highly effective for recurrent rectal cancer and, further, that the effectiveness is directly dependent upon the extent of the surgical resection: if the tumor is unresectable, the tumor control rate at 2 years is only approximately 25%; however, it is about 40% if we are able to partially resect the tumor and 65% if we are able to completely resect the tumor.

The preoperative radiochemotherapy would consist of 45–50 Gy external beam irradiation of the pelvis with adjuvant 5-fluorouracil (5 FU) with or without leucovorin. We are convinced that the addition of 5 FU enhances the local effect of the radiation therapy, albeit, with increased risk of toxicity. We know of no other regimen that has been convincingly shown to be superior. The frequency, dose, and route of administration of the 5 FU are all factors of importance that can be tailored to the patient's individual needs. The pelvic radiation treatment should be given with high energy photons (> 10 MeV) if available. Assuming that the CT scan (preferably done with the patient in the prone treatment position) shows the disease limited to the posterior portion of the pelvis, a three-field arrangement is preferred: two wedged lateral fields mated to a posterior field. Each field should be custom shaped to match the beam profile to that of the target volume. The placement of the posterior margin of the target volume is critical. It should include the entire sacrum with a 2 cm margin, depending on the extent of posterior extension of cancer. The cephalad margin should be placed 1 cm above the sacroiliac joints. Depending on the anterior extension of cancer, the anterior margin of the target volume need not extend much more than 2–3 cm anterior to the sacral promontory. The caudal border of the target volume should extend well below the coccyx – we routinely place it just proximal to the anus [the anus and the natal cleft should be identified with radio-opaque markers (solder) at the time of simulation]. The lateral borders should encompass the sacroiliac joints with a margin of at least 1 cm.

Four to six weeks following the radiochemotherapy we would repeat the chest X-ray and abdominal-pelvic CT to assess tumor response and, more importantly, metastatic disease. In the face of advancing metastases, we would offer no further treatment other than perhaps a boost dose of 10–15 Gy to the bulk disease via custom-shaped reduced fields. But if the metastatic disease is still stable and if the patient is able and willing, we would seriously consider exploratory surgery in the specially equipped IOEBRT surgical suite. We would make every attempt to remove all gross disease, even resecting the distal two to three segments of the sacrum along with the coccyx, if necessary. To the sacral stump and the presacral hollow (presumably the tumor bed), we would deliver 10–15 Gy IOEBRT using an applicator as large as is practical.

At this point, assuming that the hepatic metastatic disease is limited to a few isolated lesions which have essentially remained stable on chemotherapy, we would favor consideration of resection of the hepatic lesions. The ones which cannot be approached surgically can be implanted intraoperatively using radioactive 125 seeds with a Mick applicator under ultrasound guidance. If the hepatic metastatic disease is such that a single large lesion is present, requiring massive liver resection, the lesion can be debulked and the tumor bed irradiated with placement of I^{125} seeds or IOEBRT. If the tumor bed happens to be at inferior vena cava's surface, I^{125} seeds can be embedded in Gelfoam (which, in turn, is wrapped in Surgicel) and the entire "patty" applied on the inferior vena cava surface by securing it with a few small sutures.

Should we, on the other hand, conclude that the patient does not have a protracted life expectancy, we would offer palliative radiochemotherapy (as described above) without IOEBRT. In general, we do not favor short, high-dose per fraction courses of radiotherapy to large target volumes in the pelvis or abdomen, as we feel that toxicity is increased by such maneuvers with little gain except convenience.

In general, treatment decisions regarding palliative care are often more complex than those regarding definitive care for the oncology patient. One must balance the risks and costs of any proposed therapy in any given situation against the expected benefits of said therapy. This can be exceedingly difficult and complicated for the responsible radiation oncologist. A multitude of factors (outlined by Dr. Kagan in his introduction to this volume) must be carefully weighed, often in an environment strained by emotions of patient and family – notably depression, anxiety and often anger. Years of clinical experience probably constitute the single most important decision making tool for palliative oncologic care. Palliative cancer care is not easy!

33 History of Lymphoma with Abnormal Magnetic Resonance Imaging

A.D. Steinfeld and J.S. Cooper

Six months ago, a 62-year-old white man had a diffuse T-cell lymphoma involving the skin of the right cheek which was successfully treated by radiations. He now presents with vertical diplopia and an inferior oblique extraocular muscle palsy. Magnetic resonance imaging (MRI) reveals abnormalities in both sides of the frontal falx and in the genu of corpus. Over the next month, he rapidly becomes confused, lethargic, and disoriented. Cerebrospinal fluid (CSF) examination is negative. Repeat MRI again shows three masses suggestive of metastases. He now has tumorous nodules on his scalp, forehead, and neck.

1. What would you recommend?
2. Would you irradiate the brain? The brain plus spinal cord?
3. Is a repeat tissue diagnosis necessary?
4. Is systemic and/or intrathecal chemotherapy indicated?
5. If patient is human immunodeficiency virus (HIV) negative or HIV positive, would your recommendations be different?
6. [Include other considerations that would influence your recommendation].

Response

Can appropriate palliative care be delivered to a patient who has rapidly evolving neurologic deterioration and no histologic diagnosis? To approach this issue, we ask several more circumscribed, component questions: Is additional investigation of his disease mandatory? What is the nature of his intracranial disease and is it related to his previously diagnosed T-cell lymphoma? Does he require biopsy of his central nervous system (CNS) lesions? How should he be treated?

Alan D. Steinfeld, MD, Jay S. Cooper, MD, New York University Medical Center, Department of Radiation Oncology, 566 First Avenue, New York, NY 10016, USA

How Much Investigation Is Enough?

In nearly all instances, tissue diagnosis is a prerequisite to therapy; different treatment may be required for different kinds of tumors or histologically identical tumors of varying extent. However, exceptions exist. They are justified by the principle that biopsy should be deferred when the risk of obtaining a specimen exceeds the value of having the information that a histologic diagnosis would provide. In this case, the description of the lesions (on both sides of the frontal falx and in the genu) suggests that tissue could be obtained reasonably safely. But, is biopsy required or is the situation sufficiently clear to permit the construction of a plan of action without a histologic specimen? A somewhat more subtle issue relates to how many different lesions should be biopsied in the same patient. It is generally unreasonable and unnecessary to biopsy every metastatic lesion that a patient develops. Rather, the inherent biologic behavior of each type of cancer determines the likelihood that any subsequent lesion is related to previously detected tumor. For example, we would accept a typical-appearing, contrast-enhancing, intra-cerebral lesion in a patient who had pre-existent metastatic lung or breast tumor as another manifestation of the metastatic process; we would not so readily accept a radiographically identical appearing lesion as similarly metastatic in a patient who had metastatic prostate cancer. In the formed instance, CNS metastases are common, in the latter rare. Thus, we must ask how likely would a cutaneous T-cell lymphoma be associated with subsequent cerebral disease? If we have enough data to answer these questions with a reasonable degree of certainly, biopsy may be unnecessary.

Nature of the Intracranial Disease

We are told nothing about the MRI appearance of the cerebral lesions, only their approximate location. We must consider the possibility that they are neoplastic or infectious (we assume they are not artifactual), and the possibility that more than one process is occurring simultaneously.

Let us consider non-neoplastic etiologies first. In current practice, it is difficult not to think of acquired immunodeficiency syndrome (AIDS) in any patient who has cerebral lesions and rapidly progressive deterioration. Sixty-two years is somewhat older than most patients who have AIDS, but not sufficiently so to persuade us to discount the possibility. The patient's history of a prior lymphoma may initially raise our suspicions; but, the findings are not suggestive of AIDS because of the T-cell nature of the prior disease (nearly all AIDS-associated lymphomas are of B-cell lineage). If we knew that the patient was infected by HIV, infectious explanations of his neurologic problems would become more likely. A variety of infections can produce the symptoms noted in this patient, and can coexist with CNS lymphoma, particularly in an immunocompromised host. For example, infection by cytomegalovirus or HIV itself can account for this patient's neurologic symptoms. However, the mass lesions observed on MRI are not suggestive of these infections. Nonviral infections can produce space occupying abnormalities on scan (McCormack et al. 1990), and are a more plausible diagnostic consideration in this man. The most common of these infections in patients who have AIDS is toxoplasmosis. MRI and computed tomography (CT) may be suggestive in distinguishing toxoplasmosis from primary CNS lymphoma (Kupfer et al. 1990; Dina 1991). Toxoplasmosis tends to present as multifocal lesions of the white or deep-gray matter and white–gray interface, while primary CNS lymphoma typically involves the white matter, sparing the deep-gray matter. Additionally, primary CNS lymphoma lesions tend to be fewer in number and larger than "toxo" lesions. The findings in this patient therefore are more suggestive of lymphoma than toxoplasmosis.

Other infectious etiologies include fungal abscesses (*Cryptococcus* neoforms being the most common) or bacterial abscesses, but there is no compelling reason to invoke these possibilities in this patient other than the ill-defined immunosuppressive associated with the development of lymphoma. Had the patient required aggressive cytotoxic chemotherapy for his prior lymphoma, we would be more suspicious.

A previously well-controlled problem, tuberculosis, is again becoming a major health threat. We have seen a small number of patients who had similar clinical histories and abnormal scans but who on biopsy were found to have cerebral tuberculosis. However, such speculation seems to us unwarranted in this patient who we have no particular reason to suspect is infected by HIV. Possible neoplastic diagnoses that we would consider for this patient include intracranial spread of his known T-cell lymphoma, primary CNS lymphoma (PCNSL), other primary CNS neoplasms (e.g., gliomas) and metastatic tumors from an as yet undetected primary source. Information regarding the MRI appearance of the lesions and response to administration of contrast material (e.g., gadolinium) is not supplied. We are also not told if a CT scan was done. If the tumors were round, well-marginated and contrast-enhancing, their appearance would support the diagnosis of metastases from a solid tumor. However, nothing in the supplied case report suggests another source of origin (e.g., a primary lung cancer or melanoma) unrelated to this T-cell lymphoma, and we, therefore, consider this possibility too remote to warrant further discussion. A primary glioma is consistent with the patient's age, but unlikely based upon the multiplicity of lesions seen on MRI.

We therefore arrive at the conclusion that the patient likely has lymphomatous involvement of this CNS and now must decide whether it is related to his previously diagnosed T-cell lymphoma. The idea that the prior cutaneous lesion on his cheek represents spread from a PCNSL is mentioned only to be rejected, as metastases outside the CNS from such lesions are rare (Karlsson et al. 1992). While the age of the patient, multiple lesions and involvement of the corpus callosum are consistent with the diagnosis of PCNSL (DeAngelis et al. 1987), this diagnosis implies that the patient has a "new lymphoma" because virtually all PCNSL are of B-cell origin while this patient's prior biopsy indicated T-cell disease.

Systemic lymphoma that spreads to the brain usually presents as meningeal disease, rather than discrete lesions (Pagani et al. 1981; Zimmerman 1990; Aabo and Walbom-Jorgensen 1986). The abnormalities described in this patient's case report support the idea of diffuse intracerebral disease since the locations of the lesions described on MRI do not explain his ocular deficits. The description of rapidly evolving confusion, lethargy and disorientation is also suggestive of meningeal disease. In addition, the presence of tumorous nodules on his forehead, scalp, and neck suggest that his previously diagnosed lymphoma is again active and therefore offers further support for our hypothesis that the patient's systemic lymphoma has recurred and has spread to his brain. If we were to learn that the patient was infected by HIV, our conclusion would be unaltered because of the high incidence of CNS spread from systemic lymphoma in AIDS (LOUREIRO et al. 1988).

The one finding that remains "unexplained" in this context is the "negative" CSF examination. Since meningeal involvement is so common in such patients, a truly normal CSF examination is unusual. We are not told, however, how many times the CSF was sampled and precisely what was evaluated. While some series suggest that only approximately one patient in four who has lymphomatous meningitis has detectable abnormal cells in his CSF (DEANGELIS et al. 1987), elevated protein levels are evident in most patients. If we were permitted only one diagnostic maneuver in this patient, we would favor repeat analysis of the CSF. If lymphomatous cells were detected, our working diagnosis of systemic lymphoma with spread to the CNS would be confirmed and additional work-up to initiate therapy would be unnecessary.

If, however, repeat CSF analysis remains "negative," we would consider biopsy of one of the cerebral lesions. Despite literature reports that describe cerebral mass lesions occurring in patients who have systemic lymphoma, we would not be totally convinced our diagnosis was accurate if the CSF were repeatedly totally normal. Biopsy of the tumorous nodules on his skin would not be a suitable substitute in our opinion. We would assume they represent recurrence of the previously established T-cell lymphoma.

Treatment of the CNS

For the moment, we will assume that repeat CSF examination, or biopsy will establish the diagnosis of secondary, T-cell lymphoma. Questions to be considered at this juncture are:

1. What is the intention of treatment?
2. Is radiotherapy appropriate?
3. What volume should the radiotherapy field encompass?
4. What dose should be given?
5. Should systemic therapy be given?
6. What is the role of intrathecal treatment?

As might be expected of a case history in this volume, the patient's condition is beyond cure at this point. In most series, the average survival of patients who have meningeal spread of systemic lymphoma (including T-cell lymphoma) is very short. For example, SENTIS et al. (1986) observed that patients who had CNS involvement from cutaneous T-cell lymphoma had an average survival of 8 weeks (range 1–17 weeks) following diagnosis despite treatment. Thus, our intentions for this patient must be confined to palliation of the distress caused by his neurologic deterioration. And, there is a reasonable likelihood that we will be able to accomplish this with radiotherapy. LISTER et al. (1979) noted complete response to radiotherapy in all four patients treated for intracerebral deposits of metastatic lymphoma. The situation for lymphomatous meningitis was not as favorable, with only four of ten patients showing resolution of symptoms and at least partial relief of cranial nerve dysfunction. Typically, the cranial meninges down to C2 are included within the treatment portal. The tumorous nodules on his forehead and scalp should be included in the portal, thereby providing for their local control without adding toxicity. The lesion on the neck is likely to be outside the portal and we would not seek to treat it unless it produced distressing symptoms. One could consider craniospinal irradiation; however, we would choose not to do so. The systemic nature of the patient's disease argues for a systemic approach to treatment. In that the required chemotherapy will require adequate bone marrow support, we have generally not treated such patients with spinal irradiation because of the myelosuppression that it is likely to induce. Rather, we would rely upon intrathecal chemotherapy, probably delivered from an Ommaya reservoir.

Because of the limited intentions of treatment, we would seek to deliver the shortest course of treatment that would likely fulfill our objectives without unduly occupying the patient's time. In practical terms, a course of 3000 cGy delivered in ten fractions over 2 weeks meets our requirement.

Treating in the Absence of a Clear Diagnosis

This case primarily is illustrative of the thought processes inherent in designing a plan of action before a histologic diagnosis is available. A variety of other clinical situations also warrant initiating radiotherapy without confirmation of tumor and at times, without the prospect of such confirmation ever being obtained. Some of the clinical situations which we consider valid for such treatment include:

1. Multiple symptomatic CNS lesions with clinical and/or radiographic evidence of a primary tumor that frequently gives rise to CNS metastases (e.g., breast, lung)
2. Pancreatic or biliary tract lesions not amenable to biopsy
3. Airway obstruction by intrinsic tumor which cannot be biopsied because of the risk of bleeding
4. Superior vena caval obstruction with sufficiently high venous pressure that an attempt at obtaining tissue is contraindicated
5. Infiltrating brain stem tumor

The current case is not so clear cut in our minds. We would optimally prefer tissue diagnosis. However, if repeat CSF examination in this patient were to remain "negative" and if the patient's general condition or his refusal of biopsy precluded tissue diagnosis, we would (after appropriate discussion with the patient) offer him empiric therapy in light of the high likelihood that he has CNS involvement from systemic lymphoma. In most instances we would expect to be correct. We realize that occasionally we will be wrong. However, we believe that patients are best served if treatment is delivered on an empiric basis whenever the risk of medical testing exceeds the value of the information gained.

References

Aabo K, Walbom-Jorgensen S (1986) Central nervous system complications by malignant lymphomas: radiation schedule and treatment results. Int J Radiat Oncol Biol Phys 12: 197–202

Deangelis LM, Yahalom J, Rosenblum M, Posner JB (1987) Primary CNS lymphoma: managing patients with spontaneous and AIDS-related disease. Oncology 1: 52–62

Dina T (1991) Primary central nervous system lymphoma vs toxoplasmosis in AIDS. Radiology 179: 823–828

Karlsson UL, Leibel SA, Wallner K, Davis LW, Brady LW (1992) Brain. In: Perez CA, Brady LW (eds) Principles and practice of radiation oncology, 2nd edn. Lippincott, Philadelphia, pp 5436–5544

Kupfer MC, Zee CS, Colletti PM, Boswell WD, Rhodes R (1990) MRI evaluation of AIDS-related encephalopathy: toxoplasmosis vs lymphoma. Magn Reson Imaging 8: 51–57

Lister TA, Sutcliffe SBJ, Brearley RL, Cullen MH (1979) Patterns of CNS involvement in malignant lymphoma. In: Whitehouse JMA, Kay HEM (eds) CNS complications of malignant disease. University Park, Baltimore pp 131–141

Loureiro C, Gill PS, Meyer PR, Rhodes R, Rarick MU, Levine AM (1988) Autopsy findings in AIDS-related lymphoma. Cancer 62: 735–739

McCormack B, Cooper PR, Louie E, Koslow M (1990) Management of intracranial mass lesions in AIDS patients. Contemp Neurosurg 12: 1–6

Pagani JJ, Libshitz HI, Wallace S, Hayman LA (1981) Central nervous system leukemia and lymphoma: computed tomographic manifestations. AJR 137: 1195–1201

Sentis HJ, Padberg G, Buruma OJS, Bots GTHAM, Willemze R, Van Vloten WA (1986) Neurological complications in patients with cutaneous T-cell lymphoma. Br J Dermatol 114: 359–366

Zimmerman RA (1990) Central nervous system lymphomas. Radiol Clin North Am 28: 697–721

34 Palliative Radiation for Pulmonary Widespread Disease

O.M. Salazar and M. Suntharalingam

A 41-year-old woman had an adrenal carcinoma removed 2 years ago and was subsequently put on chemotherapy for liver metastases which failed. She then underwent a partial hepatectomy. One morning she coughed two cups of blood, and a bronchoscopy showed blood coming from the basal segment of the right lower lobe. Chest radiographs showed widespread pulmonary metastases with a large mass in the medial segment of the right lower lobe.

1. Will radiations be likely to stop hemoptysis in this situation?
2. Will it shrink the tumor that is bleeding in the right lower lobe?
3. Have you had any experience with patients with other endocrine tumors (e.g., carcinoid) in a similar situation?
4. Would you have irradiated the liver? Under what circumstances? Dose? Volume?
5. [Include other considerations that would influence your recommendation].

Response

The most recent statistics indicate that up to two-thirds of all cancer patients will receive radiation at some time during the course of their ailment. While radiation therapy plays a major role in the primary management of many different tumors, it enjoys even a wider and very firmly established role in the palliation of metastatic disease. Consistently, various radiation techniques have proven capable of achieving significant levels of symptomatic relief palliation. These impressive results have prompted oncologists to try to expand the role of radiation in a wide variety of clinical situations. Through a preselected case, in this dissertation, we are faced with the challenge of attempting to launch an accurate description of the role that ionizing radiation plays in a specific palliative setting.

Omar M. Salazar, MD, Mohan Suntharalingam, MD, University of Maryland Medical Center, Department of Radiation Oncology, 22 South Greene Street, Baltimore, MD 21201 USA

The case presented is that of a 41-year-old woman with adrenal carcinoma. She underwent a surgical resection 2 years prior and was subsequently placed on chemotherapy for liver metastases. However, this therapy also failed and she then underwent a partial hepatectomy. One morning she is found coughing up large amounts of blood. Let us assume that an emergent bronchoscopy reveals the bleeding to be originating from a lesion in the bronchial wall which is eroding into the surrounding tissues without obvious large vessel invasion. Chest X-rays show widespread pulmonary metastases together with a large mass within the medial segment of the right lower lobe.

This particular clinical situation raises a number of key questions which a radiation oncologist must answer when deciding on the use of palliative radiation therapy. Specifically, we are being asked to consider treating a large lung mass in the face of widespread disease.

Prior to the initiation of any therapy, one must have a full understanding of the objectives of the therapeutic plan. In each clinical situation, there must be well defined goals and a sound rationale for the institution of any treatment modality. In order to accomplish this one must ask a number of key questions. Is this a life-threatening situation? What are the therapeutic alternatives? What is the likelihood of obtaining the desired response? What therapeutic technique should be employed? What side effects should be expected?

Lung tumors (either primary or metastatic) can occur anywhere throughout the lung parenchyma or tracheobronchial tree. Depending on the location of the lesion, a variety of emergent clinical situations can occur. Intrinsic lesions within the bronchial lumen can lead to hemoptysis, airway obstruction, secondary infection, and/or pain. Extrinsic compression from parenchymal tumors can cause major blood vessel obstruction (i.e., superior vena cava syndrome). Submucosal tumor spread (i.e., small-cell lung cancer) can cause airway obstruction and other related problems. Direct tumor extension can lead to a tracheoesophageal fistula, cord compression, chest wall invasion and even cardiac tamponade. The judicious use of palliative radiation therapy has proven to be quite successful in many of these circumstances.

When faced with a 41-year-old patient who presents with a life-threatening situation, the oncologist must act quickly and decisively. Younger patients deserve an aggressive use of palliative radiation therapy. Radiation offers her an excellent chance of controlling the hemorrhage and improving her general level of comfort. In this circumstance these endpoints represent legitimate therapeutic goals. Palliative radiation treatment will not change the fatal course of her advanced disease. Nevertheless, while these patients will eventually succumb to their disease, the use of palliative radiation in an indicated clinical setting will certainly help to improve the quality of their lives.

In order to determine the efficacy of the therapy, one must consider a number of key factors. The histology of the lesion may provide information concerning the radioresponsiveness of the tumor. Adrenal carcinoma is an extremely rare tumor. A review of the available literature does provide some support for use of radiation in both an adjuvant as well as palliative setting (HENLEY et al. 1983). The most common sites of metastatic spread from these tumors have been reported as bone, brain and lymphatics (KING and LACK 1979). Authors have reported good symptomatic responses of metastatic adrenal carcinoma with palliative doses of external radiation (30–40 cGy) (MARKOE et al. 1991).

Because we are dealing with an adenocarcinoma, one might expect to see a more gradual radiographic regression of the lesion after treatment. It is important to remember that this does not represent radioresistance, but instead it is simply a reflection of the biologic growth/regression rate of this particular tumor cell type. An extensive personal experience with various lung cancer cell types and different radiation schedules indicate that adenocarcinoma has a very long cell doubling time and hence it represents a slower radioresponsive tumor (SALAZAR et al. 1976). This is an important point to keep in mind when attempting to quantitatively document a response to therapy since it may also be responsible for a more gradual regression of some of the patient's symptoms. One can partially overcome these basic biologic differences with the use of appropriate dose rate schedules and radiation delivery systems.

Radiation therapy has been used to achieve bleeding from advanced cervical carcinoma and esophageal varices has proven that radiation is extremely effective in the emergent setting. The biologic response to our therapy can be directly correlated to the size of the blood vessels located within the treatment field. Larger vessels have proven to be more resistant to the effects of ionizing radiation (RHEE 1986). Basic radiobiologic research has provided an explanation for this difference in sensitivity.

It is postulated that the difference is primarily due to the presence of smooth muscle within the walls of large vessels. These cells represent a fixed postmitotic cell population which, by definition, are highly differentiated and have lost their ability to divide (RUBIN and CASARET 1968). As long as they are maintained in their quiescent phase, they will not be susceptible to radiation-induced damage.

Endothelial cells represent the acutely responding tissue within the vascular system. These cells are classified as vegetative intermitotic cells which, by definition, possess a rapid cell cycling time (RUBIN and CASARET 1968). Exposure to radiation causes proliferation and sloughing of these endothelial cells which can lead to blockage of the lumen. Doses of 1200 cGy given in three fractions produces profound effects in the microvasculature within the treatment field. These changes help to produce a clinical response within 24–48 h.

Based on the responses which have been observed and reported, we believe that there is ample evidence to support the decision to initiate therapy to the lung in this specific case. Many authors have published results of the use of radiation for palliation in lung tumors. The University of Maryland experience with 568 patients treated with external beam therapy demonstrated that 86% of patients treated with hemoptysis as a presenting symptom noted rapid relief after undergoing therapy (SLAWSON and SCOTT 1979). Other reports support this study and, in fact, hemoptysis has proven to be the most responsive clinical symptom in lung tumors (SEYDEL et al. 1975).

The effects on the lung parenchyma must be considered when designing the radiation treatment portals. As an intermediate response system, the lung will display early degenerative "pneumonitic" changes as well as a chronic fibrotic phase. Adjacent structures (i.e., trachea and esophagus) can also react to radiation. Clinically, these changes may be manifested early on as dyspnea, cough and dysphagia. If the volume of irradiated tissue is too large, pulmonary scarring can lead to debilitating respiratory compromise. All radiation-induced side effects are volume, total dose, and dose rate-related phenomena.

It is important to limit the amount of normal tissue irradiated within the target volume. In the palliative setting there is no need to include draining lymphatics or to have wide margins around the area of interest. However, one must clearly define the areas responsible for the immediate clinical presentation as well as those sites which may cause problems in the future. If possible, these areas should be included in the treatment field. Clinical judgement is crucial because if these sites are initially excluded, one might be faced with the difficulty of having to consider further therapy in the midst of previously irradiated tissue. In this particular situation our patient has multiple diffuse lung metastases. Since there is no other evidence of impending obstruction or erosion, a treatment field should encompass only the lesion found to be responsible for the patient's emergent clinical presentation.

The bronchoscopy findings can help clarify the clinical situation. One must be able to accurately define the source of bleeding in order to determine the probability of instituting effective therapy. If the lesion had eroded into a major vessel then emergent radiation would not be adequate therapy to stop the bleeding. However, if there was evidence of oozing from submucosal growth of the lesion, then the bleeding may very well be controlled with emergent therapy.

The treatment of superior vena cava syndrome has provided a large body of information regarding dose tolerance to the lung. Work by Rubin and colleagues at the University of Rochester, first with animals and then in humans, has shown that daily doses of 400 cGy in three fractions can be tolerated by limited lung volumes (Rubin et al. 1963). We would recommend initially delivering these higher fractions in order to create more acute reactions within the treatment field. Once a clinical response is obtained, then it would be most prudent to lower the daily fraction size to 180–200 cGy. A total dose of 4000 cGy is adequate for a lung lesion when palliation is the aim.

When considering the doses of external beam radiation therapy, a physician is limited by the tolerances of surrounding normal tissues. If palliation is the aim, then endobronchial brachytherapy may achieve the same clinical responses with less associated morbidity. The radiation effect is limited to an isolated portion of normal bronchial tissues. Since these cells represent a postmitotic system, they are considered relatively radioresistant. This allows the application of a locally intensified dose to the area of known tumor involvement. With the ability to increase the dose with a single treatment fraction, one would expect to see a more immediate resolution of hemoptysis, airway obstruction and cough.

Clinical trials from the Christie Hospital in Manchester, UK, looked at the effectiveness of single dose brachytherapy for advanced endobronchial cancers. They prescribed 1500–2000 cGy to an area 1 cm away from the source. Symptomatic relief was assessed 6 weeks after the application. In patients presenting with hemoptysis, 86% obtained symptomatic relief. More impressively, only 18% required further therapy for recurrent symptoms (Stout 1992). Currently this institution is conducting a randomized study to compare intraluminal therapy versus external beam therapy with 3000 cGy in eight fractions for the alleviation of respiratory symptoms (Stout 1992).

With this particular patient, the situation may have arisen in which a radiation oncologist may have been asked to consider palliative liver irradiation. The same principles will apply. What would be the aim of this treatment? What are the alternatives? How would the treatment be given? What side effects may be encountered? Metastatic liver disease can give rise to acute biliary obstruction and subsequent liver failure. More often, it gives pain by distention of Glisson's capsule. This discomfort can be unbearable in a patient who has not responded to other therapies. Each of these circumstances will merit the use of radiation as a last measure. The liver tolerance is of issue since it should not exceed 3000 cGy. The radiation schedule should be short and treatment fields should be limited to the problematic areas.

The role of radiation therapy in cancer palliation is firmly established. The judicious use of this treatment can achieve significant levels of symptomatic relief and hence, improvement in the quality of life of these unfortunate patients. Radiation therapy is an alternative that should not be denied and in many instances should be utilized before it becomes hopeless to secure these endpoints.

References

Henley DJ et al. (1983) Adrenal cortical carcinoma – a continuing challenge. Surgery 6: 926–931

King DR, Lack EE (1979) Adrenal cortical carcinoma: a clinical and pathologic study of 49 cases. Cancer 44: 239–244

Markoe AM et al. (1991) Radiation therapy for adjunctive treatment of adrenal cortical carcinoma. Am J Clin Oncol 14(2): 170–174

Rhee JG (1986) The clonegenic response of bovine aortic endothelial cells in culture irradiation. Radiat Res 106: 182–189

Rubin P, Green J, Holzwasser G, Gerle R (1963) Superior vena caval syndrome: slow dose versus rapid high dose schedules. Radiology, 81: 388 – 401

Rubin R, Casaret GW (1968) Clinical radiation pathology, vol 1. Saunders, Philadelphia

Salazar OM, Rubin P, Brown JC, Feldstein ML, Keller B (1976) Predictors of radiation response in lung cancer: a clinical pathobiological analysis. Cancer 37(6): 2636–2650

Seydel HG, Chait A, Gmelich JT (1975) Cancer of the lung. Wiley, New York, pp 158–164

Slawson RG, Scott RM (1979) Radiation therapy in bronchogenic carcinoma. Radiology, 132(1): 175–176

Stout R (1992) Single dose brachytherapy for endobronchial cancer. International brachytherapy programme and abstracts, 7th International brachytherapy working conference, Nucletron International, Wageninger, Netherlands (Chap. 22)

35 Symptomatic Multiple Cerebral Lesions

L.R. PROSNITZ

A 70-year-old white woman presented with progressive weakness in her lower left extremity and mental confusion. Computed tomography (CT) revealed a hemorrhagic mass in the right frontal lobe. Magnetic resonance imaging (MRI) showed three additional cerebral lesions which resembled metastases or infarcts. A metastatic work-up was otherwise negative. The patient's symptoms improved somewhat on Decadron.

1. Would you irradiate the brain without a tissue diagnosis?
2. What is the differential diagnosis?
3. Was a metastatic work-up necessary? To find the primary? To find other metastases?
4. What is your estimate of survival and quality of survival?
5. [Include other considerations that would influence your recommendation].

Response

The case described raises two substantive issues: (1) whether to treat on the presumption of a diagnosis of malignancy without actually obtaining histologic proof, and (2) the appropriate evaluation and management of a patient who presents with presumed metastatic disease without a known primary lesion. If asked to see such a patient in consultation with a history approximately as outlined in the case report, I would proceed as follows:

I would first assess the clinical probability of the diagnosis of metastatic carcinoma. The history is a bit lacking in detail that would help to differentiate vascular disease in the brain from metastases. Was the onset of neurologic symptoms progressive over short or longer period of time? Are there other factors in the past history that suggest a high-risk of cerebral vascular disease, such as vascular disease elsewhere or hypertension? What is the confidence of the neuroradiologist in the diagnosis of either metastatic disease or vascular lesions? Some symptomatic improvement with Decadron (dexamethasone) would be expected with either diagnosis and is not terribly helpful in distinguishing between the two.

Although one can probably make a clinical diagnosis of metastatic disease with greater than 90% accuracy, nonetheless, histologic confirmation is highly desirable if not mandatory in almost all instances and with the use of the newer stereotactic biopsy techniques should be achievable with minimum morbidity (COIA 1992). One should always be extremely cautious about making a diagnosis of a fatal illness (metastatic carcinoma to the brain) without histologic proof.

Let us assume that the clinical history, CT and MRI findings of the brain are most compatible with the diagnosis of metastatic disease and that histologic confirmation has indeed been obtained. The cryptic comment in the case report that a "metastatic work-up was otherwise negative" begs the issues. At our institution, such a patient in the great majority of instances would receive a full metastatic evaluation including, for example, CT scans of the chest, abdomen, and pelvis, barium studies of the gastrointestinal (GI) tract, bone scan, in perverse defiance of the published literature on the subject which indicates such a work-up to be of little value in the great majority of instances. At the other extreme we have seen patients in the circumstances described in this case report go promptly to neurosurgical exploration without so much as having a chest X-ray.

In our judgement, the proper course of action is a limited, focused, cost-effective evaluation for metastatic disease with emphasis on the detection and recognition of treatable entities. This evaluation begins with review of the histopathology. The group at Vanderbilt has recently drawn attention to the en-tity of poorly differentiated carcinoma and poorly differentiated adenocarci-

Leonard R. Prosnitz, MD, Department of Radiation Oncology, Duke University Medical Center, Box 3085–154, Durham, NC 27710, USA

noma of unknown primary site (GRECO and HAINSWORTH 1992; HAINSWORTH et al. 1992). This is an uncommon subset of patients with metastatic malignancies of unknown primary site, comprising about 20% of the total and occurring mostly in younger patients under the age of 50 years. It is, however, a highly treatable subset with a small percentage of patients apparently cured of their malignancy with aggressive platinum-based combination chemotherapy.

The evaluation would further include, of course, a history and physical examination with special attention to smoking history, exam of breasts, thyroid, pelvis and rectum. Appropriate laboratory studies outside the central nervous system (CNS) would include chest film, mammograms, stool guaiac exam, prostate-specific antigen and other tests as may be suggested by specific symptoms. Apart from poorly differentiated malignancies it is also quite useful to detect breast or prostate carcinoma as a primary site for the metastases, but they are both quite unusual as a source for metastatic carcinoma of unknown origin (ULTMAN 1991).

I believe it is appropriate to find those metastatic malignancies for which effective treatment is available and/or those that can be found quite easily. In other instances it isn't worth the trouble. Unfortunately the number of metastatic malignancies that can be effectively treated are few in number. It has been repeatedly demonstrated that the administration of chemotherapy for the great majority of solid metastatic tumors is of no value in improving survival and of questionable value in achieving palliation. There is no evidence that early detection and treatment of metastatic malignancies is of value. The diseases that can be readily treated and that one would like to detect include breast, prostate and thyroid, all of which may be responsive to hormonal manipulations of one sort or another. For the great majority of solid tumors such as lung, colorectal, upper GI, renal we have only very limited chemotherapy available. There is little point in early detection of metastatic disease in these tumors and frankly not much point to systemic chemotherapy outside of the study setting. If one does detect a primary lesion a search for other metastases is similarly of very little value.

All of these comments apply to asymptomatic patients. If a patient is having bone pain, for example, it is certainly of value to detect metastatic disease thay may be causing that pain and treat accordingly. Similarly specific symptomatology that may be related to local disease any place should be investigated and its cause determined if possible so that appropriate local regional treatment (usually radiation) can be administered. In the asymptomatic patient, however, little is to be gained by early detection of metastatic disease.

It is worth doing simple things like a chest X-ray to diagnose a metastatic lung carcinoma. An abnormal chest film may provide a more accessible site to biopsy than the brain. It is useful to end speculation as to the source of the primary lung lesion, if this can be simply and easily done with something such as a chest X-ray.

In general, in this era of the ability to biopsy many sites of the body with radiographic assistance and little morbidity and difficulty, I would not treat this patient or hardly any other patient without a tissue diagnosis. In the case described, stereotactic brain biopsy would appear to be indicated. In our institution this is usually carried out with very little difficulty. If a lesion should present itself on chest X-ray, I would biopsy that lesion first and accept that as histologic confirmation of the brain process, provided the neuroradiologists were reasonably confident in the diagnosis of metastatic disease.

The majority of patients with metastatic malignancies of unknown origin will have an epidermoid or adenocarcinoma that is not poorly differentiated and that is unresponsive to treatment (SPORN and GREENBERG 1990). Survival is very poor with approximately 50% of patients over the age of 50 dead in 3–7 months. Oncologists should emphasize quality of life for these patients and not spend their few remaining months in lengthy diagnostic and/or therapeutic endeavors that are highly unlikely to be of any benefit.

My approach to treatment would be as follows: Assume that histologic confirmation of metastatic disease in the brain has been confirmed and that no primary site is evident elsewhere. The patient needs whole brain radiation. The aggressiveness of this therapy should be influenced by the patient's overall condition and histology of the metastatic process. If the patient's general condition was good apart from her neurologic problems and I felt there was a reasonable chance of survival beyond 6 months, I would tend to treat with daily fractions of about 200 cGy to a total dose of 4400 cGy. If the metastatic disease were relatively limited in volume in the brain, I would consider boosting a small area of the brain for an additional 600–1000 cGy. If the patient's general condition was not particularly good, more rapid fractionation would be appropriate, such as

3000 cGy in ten fractions. The latter treatment scheme has been standard practice for many years, but has become less popular recently because of concerns of long-term neurologic damage that might result from the use of high fraction radiation. Such damage has been usually in patients receiving chemotherapy as well as radiation for diseases such as small cell lung cancer. We do know, however, that large fractions greater than 200 cGy are more prone to cause late normal tissue reactions compared with fraction of 200 cGy or less. I think the 200 cGy approach is now used too often rather than too little but do recommend it for the circumstances described above.

References

Coia LR (1992) The role of radiation therapy in the treatment of brain metastases. Int J Radiat Oncol Biol Phys 23: 229–238

Greco FA, Hainsworth JD (1992) Tumors of unknown origin. Cancer 42: 96–115

Hainsworth JD, Johnson DH, Greco FA (1992) Cisplatin-based combination chemotherapy in the treatment of poorly differentiated carcinoma and poorly differentiated adenocarcinoma of unknown primary site: results of a 12-year experience. J Clin Oncol 10: 912–922

Ultman JE (1991) Cancer of unknown primary site. Cancer Res Clin Oncol 117: 505–509

Sporn JR, Greenberg BR (1990) Emperic chemotherapy in patients with carcinoma of unknown primary site. Am J Med 88: 49–55

36 Multiple Cancers and Diffuse Bony Metastases

D.Y. Tong

Twelve years ago, a man who is now 81 years old had stage II adenocarcinoma of the left breast managed by radical mastectomy. Ten years ago, he had a well-differentiated adenocarcinoma of the prostate, stage A1, treated by irradiation. He now has fatigue with pain in his left shoulder and back. Imaging studies show a large excavating mass in the right lower lobe of the lung extending to the pleura with a large effusion. Lytic and blastic lesions are seen in the thoracic and lumbar spine and the right acetabula. Bone scan reveals increased uptake in the ribs bilaterally and in the left hemipelvis. A homogeneously enlarged prostate has been found with a prostate-specific antigen (PSA) level of 5.25, elevated serum alkaline phosphatase, and a hemoglobin of 10 g/dl.

1. How would you manage the pleural effusion? Osseous metastases?
2. What is the differential diagnosis?
3. Do you need histologic confirmation before undertaking management?
4. [Include other considerations that would influence your recommendation].

Response

This 81-year-old gentleman has widespread bony metastases, with a mixture of osteoblastic and osteolytic lesions. Both prostate cancer and breast cancer in his past can metastasize late. With a current cavitating lung lesion in his right lower lobe, extending to the pleura with a large effusion, he may well have a third party malignancy in his lung. All three cancers can spread to the bones resulting in a mixture of blastic and lytic lesions.

His prostate cancer 10 years ago was a stage A1 well-differentiated adenocarcinoma, treated with radiation therapy. Presently, the prostate gland is homogeneously enlarged with PSA of 5.25 ng/dl. Even though a low PSA level does not always exclude the presence of metastatic lesion, the likelihood of metastatic prostate cancer in this case remains low. Breast cancer can present with both osteoblastic and osteolytic bone metastases. A previous stage II breast cancer can certainly be a culprit in this situation. Furthermore, the bone lesions can come from heterogenous sources such as a combination of breast cancer and lung cancer.

With the advancement of modern technology, diagnostic work-up should be carefully selected in order to benefit the patient's management without undue discomfort, yet be cost effective. The patient's performance and mental status also need to be taken into account. This man obviously had a complete blood picture and blood chemistry profile to show a hemoglobin level of 10 g/dl and elevated alkaline phosphatase which are in keeping with widespread bone metastases with or without bone marrow involvement. Attention should also be paid to the serum calcium level which is sometimes elevated in patients with widespread bone metastases and lung cancer. Proper management of hypercalcemia will improve the patient's well being. A serum prostate acid phosphatase (PAP) is worth checking, as in most cases of bone metastasis from prostate cancer the PAP tends to be elevated. This may suggest whether prostate cancer is a contributing source for this patient's bone lesions. When systemic agents are used in his treatment, due consideration can be given.

For his pain in the left shoulder, plain radiography of the left shoulder region may be informative. When the lesion is mainly osteolytic, bone scan may not be positive in this area. If a lytic lesion or lesions are found in the proximal left humerus, the size of the lesion and the amount of cortical destruction will determine if prophylactic surgery is advisable to prevent a fracture. By convention, prophylactic fixation has been recommended when the lesions exceed 2.5 cm, involve 50% of the bone diameter, and invade the bone cortex (Cornell and Lane 1987).

Daphne Y. Tong, MD, Group Health Hospital, Radiation Oncology, 200 15th Avenue, East Seattle, WA 98112, USA

Fortunately, the humerus is not a weight-bearing bone, posing less danger of fracture.

The patient also has pain in his back. Careful neurological examinations should be conducted to detect any spinal cord compression by the tumor, which is one of the oncological emergencies that timely treatment is important to the patient's quality of life. Physical examination may indicate the level of cord involvement. Further radiological studies would confirm the diagnosis and the level of vertebral bodies to guide the radiation portal arrangement. Myelogram with metrizamide, computed tomography (CT) and magnetic resonance imaging (MRI) have all been useful, yet the sensitivity and noninvasive nature of MRI renders it the most appropriate study for these elderly patients (Aichner et al. 1987). In the presence of spinal cord compression, which is most often extradural, radiation therapy combined with steroids should start as soon as possible. The radiation portal includes the site of spinal cord involvement and generally extends two vertebral bodies above and below the site of compression (Kornblith and Cassady 1985). Parallel opposed anteroposterior fields are often used for the cervical and lumbar regions, while posterior field alone is often used for the thoracic lesions with the depth of calculation about 5–6 cm depending on the individual patient. Commonly employed doses are 3000–4000 cGy over 2–4 weeks (Kornblith and Cassady 1985). Greenberg and associates administered high-dose dexamethasone (100 mg) at diagnosis followed by high-dose radiotherapy (500 cGy for the first 3 days of treatment), then 300 cGy per day to a total dose of 3000 cGy (Greenberg et al. 1980). The results were not different from the slower dose fractionation from the same institute reported by Gilbert et al. (1978), but pain relief was substantial, probably from the steroid. During the radiotherapy course, the patient should be monitored closely for his neurological status. Surgical decompression may be indicated if there is evidence of neurological deterioration.

In the presence of a large pleural effusion, thoracentesis can serve a dual purpose of therapy and diagnosis. The fluid withdrawn is sent for bacteriologic study and cytology, as well as for chemistry to determine if the fluid is a transudate or exudate. Cytopathologic techniques would allow an experienced pathologist to recognize cancer cells in the fluid. Immunochemical techniques by assays using polyclonal sera or monoclonal antibodies are now routinely used in the diagnosis of malignancy. In this case, there should be special request for hormonal receptor studies; estrogen receptor (ER) and progesterone receptor (PR), as well as PAP and PSA. The organ specificity of PAP and PSA has resulted in their utilization by pathologists for confirmation of the prostate gland as the site of origin of metastatic tumor (Feiner and Gonzalea 1982; Allhoff et al. 1983). However, the absence of steroid receptors or PAP and PSA studies in his pleural fluid does not rule out the possibility of breast or prostate cancer in his bones. After all, by the way of presentation, the pleural effusion is most likely secondary to his lung lesion. If the cytology reveals a malignancy other than adenocarcinoma, we can conclude that the lung lesion is a third primary tumor. In case the cytology turns out to be adenocarcinoma, it is still likely to come from the peripherally located cavitating lung lesion. Whether the lung tumor is a primary or a metastatic, the management of it will not differ. If the patient develops chest pain or hemoptysis, palliative irradiation to the lung lesion should be recommended. Radiation therapy has a high success rate in relieving symptoms from lung tumors. In a retrospective analysis of patients treated for inoperable carcinoma of the lung, chest pain was controlled in 61% and hemoptysis in 84% (Slawson and Scott 1979). Unfortunately, there is no consensus or optimum dose schedule for palliative irradiation in each given situation. For this patient with advanced disease, short course external beam irradiation with a small field size covering the lung tumor is in order. The Medical Research Council in the UK instigated a sequence of prospective trials comparing 30 Gy in ten fractions against 17 Gy in two fractions, 1 week apart and 17 Gy in two fractions against 10 Gy in a single fraction for non-oat cell lung cancer. There was no difference in survival or symptom relief between the different regimens (Bleehen et al. 1990).

In the situation that the pleural fluid cytology is nondiagnostic, further pursuance with bronchoscopy or CT-guided needle biopsy of the lung tumor will be of low yield and unwarranted. Bronchoscopy is unlikely to reach the peripheral location of the tumor. Biopsy specimen from a cavitating lesion often shows necrosis only.

If the patient's pleural effusion re-accumulates after the initial thoracentesis, causing respiratory discomfort, tube thoracostomy can be done for drainage and allow the visceral pleura to come into direct contact with the parietal pleura, obliterating the pleural space. A sclerosing agent: antibiotic, antineoplastic or radioactive, can be introduced intrapleurally to produce mesothelial fibrosis (Leff et al. 1978). Various agents have been used in the past, but tetracycline has enjoyed its popularity for its consistently better results with significantly less fever and pleural chest pain (BAYLY et al. 1978; ZALOZNEK et al. 1983; O'NEILL et al. 1980; GUPTA et al. 1980). With administration of adequate analgesics, the procedure should be tolerated by this patient.

Systemic management of this patient can be challenging if the source or sources of the metastases are not certain. Nevertheless, a few considerations are worth mentioning. Chemotherapy has shown little benefit in non-small cell carcinoma of the lung. With his age and widespread bony metastases even for small cell lung carcinoma, chemotherapy may not be worth the side effects. Since breast cancer is a possible source of the bone lesions, it would be reasonable to try hormonal manipulation. It has been reported that men with advanced breast cancer respond to orchiectomy in 87% of cases and adrenalectomy in 76% (MEYSKENS et al. 1976). Not only this indicates that most male breast cancer is hormone-dependent, the majority are ER-positive and slightly less frequently PR positive (GRIFFITH and MUGGIA 1989). Even though the standard therapy has been orchiectomy, which can be performed under local anesthesia and which is beneficial for both breast and prostate cancers, tamoxifen should be tried first for physiological and psychological reasons. The response rate is expected to be better than 50% (SWAIN 1991).

A form of medical castration by using a luteinizing hormone-releasing hormone (LHRH) agonist buserelin with or without antiandrogen flutamide has been reported (VOROBIOF and FALKSON 1987; DOBERAUER et al. 1988). The nasally applied buserelin is associated with tolerable side effects such as hot flashes and impotence. If the patient has active prostate cancer, this treatment modality would also be appropriate.

If the patient's bone pain is not relieved by analgesics, radiation therapy to the painful bone lesions is effective in pain relief, reduction of the need for narcotics, improving ambulation and even arrest of local tumor growth. Results from a multicenter study showed 80%–90% with partial pain relief and 50% with complete relief (TONG et al. 1982). The sites of metastases have not been shown to correlate with the degree of pain relief. Whether the patient's bone lesions are from the breast, prostate or lung in origin, he has a good chance of being palliated.

The patient's life expectancy is certainly limited. Effective treatment with minimal morbidity over as short a time span as possible would be ideal. From the original report of the Radiation Therapy Oncology Group (RTOG) study, variety of dose-fractionation schedules were used (TONG et al. 1982). No significant difference in response was noted. A subsequent re-analysis of the data suggested that the protracted fractionation schemes (270 cGy in 15 fractions, or 300 cGy in ten fractions) were more effective (BLITZER 1985). A few retrospective studies of multiple fractionation to 2000–4000 cGy versus single fraction 400–1500 cGy failed to show a striking difference between the two treatment regimens (VARGHA et al. 1969; PENN 1976; GARMATIS and CHU 1978). Other prospective randomized studies supported the view that effective pain relief could be achieved with single fraction or short course radiation therapy (COLE 1989; MADESN 1983). With the controversy of dose-fractionation and the lack of consensus, the radiation oncologist must consider the site of disease, the tolerance of the normal tissue in the radiation field, the patient's performance status and social situation in deciding upon a suitable treatment regimen.

Other methods of palliative radiation, such as hemibody irradiation and systemic radioisotopes can be considered if the pain is diffuse throughout the bony skeleton. Sequential hemibody irradiation is designed to spare the patient with multiple sites of metastatic disease from repeated trips for radiation. Salazar reported complete and partial pain relief of 21% and 77% respectively in this study with most of the patients having cancers of the breast, prostate or lung (SALAZAR et al. 1986). Pain control was achieved promptly with half of them improving within 2 days. Patients treated to the upper of hemibody were hospitalized for 1 day for hydration and premedication with antiemetics and corticosteroids. The dose was 600 cGy midplane. Patients receiving mid- and lower-body treatments were given 800 cGy, and were premedicated as outpatients for nausea and vomiting. He found that the pain relief was long lasting and without the need of retreatment for at least 50% of the remaining patients' lives. The combination of hemibody irradiation in conjunction with local field irradiation for bone metastases has been explored. Recently completed RTOG 82–06 study compared local field radiation therapy (300 cGy in ten fractions) to local field plus hemibody irradiation (single dose 800 cGy). For those patients surviving long enough to allow observation, the time to disease progression, new disease and new treatment was delayed for those assigned to receive local and hemibody irradiation (POULTER et al. 1992).

Fractionated hemibody irradiation has also been reported (Tochner et al. 1982; Zelefsky et al. 1989). In Zelefsky's study, a regimen of 2500–3000 cGy in nine to ten fractions was compared with a single dose of 600 cGy or 800 cGy depending upon whether the upper or lower hemibody was irradiated. Although the median survival of both groups from the time of initial treatment was similar (10 and 11 months), the median duration for palliation was greater from those patients receiving the fractionated regimen as compared with single dose therapy (8.5 months versus 2.8 months) (Zelefsky et al. 1989) . The treatment-related toxicity was similar for both groups. A current RTOG study (88–22) is exploring the advantages of fractionated hemibody irradiation on a dose escalating schedule in patients with bony metastases from breast or prostate cancers.

Systemic radioisotopes have been used to palliate bone pain from metastatic disease. Phosphorus-32 has been given after priming the patient with testosterone or parathyroid hormones to increase uptake into neoplastic tissue (Maxfield et al. 1958; Ariel and Hassouna 1985; Aziz et al. 1986; Fowler and Whitmore 1982). However, transient exacerbation of pain, even spinal cord compression or death can occur (Fowler and Whitmore 1982). Other radioisotopes, strontium-89 (Reddy et al. 1986) and iodine-131(Eisenhut et al. 1986) have shown effectiveness with low toxicity. This modality can be reserved for failure of pain control by other methods.

We may never know the source or sources of this patient's widespread bony metastases. It is more important to manage his symptoms with sensible diagnostic work-up and carefully planned treatment with minimal toxicity. In a situation of incurable disease, augmenting the quality of life becomes the ultimate goal.

References

Aichner F, Poewe W, Rogalsky W et al. (1987) Magnetic resonance imaging in the diagnosis of spinal cord diseases. J Neurol Neurosurg Psychiatr 48: 1220

Allhoff EP, Proppe KH, Chapman CM et al. (1983) Evaluation of prostate-specific acid phosphatase and prostate-specific antigen in identification of prostate cancer. J Urol 129: 315–318

Ariel IM, Hassouna H (1985) Carcinoma of the prostate. The treatment of bone metastases by radioactive phosphorous (^{32}P). Int Surg 70: 63–66

Aziz H, Choi K, Sohn C et al. (1986) Comparison of ^{32}P therapy and sequential hemibody irradiation (HBI) for bony metastases as methods of whole body irradiation. Am J Clin Oncol 9: 264–268

Bayly TC, Kisner DL, Sybert A et al. (1978) Tetracycline and quinacrine in the control of malignant pleural effusions: a randomized trial. Cancer 41: 1188

Bleehen NM, Girling DJ, Fayers PM et al. (1990) Two consecutive controlled clinical trials of palliative radiotherapy for inoperable non small cell lung cancer (NSCLC). Proceedings of the first international consensus workshop on radiation therapy in the treatment of metastatic and locally advanced cancer. (Abstr. 3B-1)

Blitzer PH (1985) Reanalysis of the RTOG study of the palliation of symptomatic osseous metastases. Cancer 55: 1468–1472

Cole DJ (1989) A randomized trial of a single treatment versus conventional fraction in the palliative radiotherapy of painful bone metastasis. Clin Oncol 1: 59–62

Cornell CN, Lane JM (1987) Specific sites of metastatic disease and emergencies: management of pathologic fractures. In: Harris JR, Hellman S, Henderson IC, Kinne DW (eds) Breast diseases. Lippincott, Philadelphia, pp 525–532

Doberauer C, Niederle N, Schmidt CG (1988) Advanced male breast cancer treatment with the LH-RH analogue Buserelin alone or in combination with the antiandrogen flutamide. Cancer 62: 474–478

Eisenhut M, Berberich R, Kimmig B et al. (1986) Iodine-131-labelled diphosphonates for palliative treatment of bone metastases: II preliminary clinical results with Iodine-131 BPD3. J Nucl Med 27: 1255–1261

Feiner HD, Gonzalea R (1982) Carcinoma of the prostate with a typical immunohistologic features: clinical and histologic correlates. Am J Surg Pathol 10: 765–770

Fowler JE Jr, Whitmore WF Jr (1982) Consideration for the use of testosterone with systemic chemotherapy in prostate cancer. Cancer 49: 1373–1377

Garmatis CJ, Chu FCH (1978) The effectiveness of radiation therapy in the treatment of bone metastases from breast cancer. Radiology 126: 235–237

Gilbert RW, Kim JH, Posner JB (1978) Epidural spinal cord compression from metastatic tumor: diagnosis and treatment. Ann Neurol 3: 40–51

Greenberg HS, Kim JH, Posner JB (1980) Epidural spinal cord compression from metastatic tumor: results with a new treatment protocol. Ann Neurol 8: 361–366

Griffith H, Muggia FM (1989) Male breast cancer: update on systemic therapy. Reviews on Endocrine-Related Cancer 31: 5–11

Gupta N, Opfell RW, Padova C et al. (1980) Intrapleural bleomycin vs tetracycline for control of malignant pleural effusions. A randomized study. Am Soc Clin Oncol C-189: 366 (abstract)

Kornblith PL, Cassady JR (1985) Central nervous system emergencies. In: DeVita VT, Hellman S, Rosenberg SA (eds) Principles and practice of oncology. 2nd edn. Lippincott, Philadelphia, p 1960

Leff A, Honeywell PC, Costello J (1978) Pleural effusion from malignance. Ann Intern Med 88: 532

Madesn EL (1983) Painful bone metastasis: efficacy of radiotherapy assessed by the patients: a randomized trial comparing 4 Gy × 6 versus 10 Gy × 2. Int J Radiat Oncol Biol Phys 9: 1775–1779

Maxfield JR, Maxfield JJR, Maxfield WS (1958): The use of radioactive phosphorous and testosterone in metastatic bone lesions from breast and prostate. South Med J 51: 320–327

Meyskens FL, Tormey DC, Neifeld JP (1976) Male breast cancer: a review. Cancer Treat Rev 3: 83–93

O'Neill W, Spurr C, Muss H et al. (1980) A prospective study of chest tube drainage and tetracycline sclerosis versus chest tube drainage in the treatment of malignant pleural effusion. Proc Am Soc Clin Oncol 21: 349

Penn CRH (1976) Single dose and fractionated palliative irradiation for osseous metastases. Clin Radiol 29: 405–408

Poulter CA, Cosmatos D, Rubin P et al. (1992) A report of RTOG 8206: a phase III study of whether the addition of single-dose hemibody irradiation to standard fractionated local field irradiation is more effective than local field irradiation alone in the treatment of symptomatic osseous metastases. Int J Radiat Oncol Biol Phys 23: 207–214

Reddy EK, Robinson RG, Mansfield CM (1986) Strontium-89 therapy for palliation of bone metastases. J Natl Med Assoc 78: 27–32

Salazar OM, Rubin P, Hendricksoon FR et al. (1986) Single-dose half-body irradiation for palliation of multiple bone metastases from solid tumors: final radiation therapy oncology group report. Cancer 58: 29–36

Slawson RG, Scott RM (1979) Radiation therapy in bronchogenic carcinoma. Radiology 132: 175–176

Swain SM (1991) Review of the article "Management of male breast cancer." Oncology 5(3): 47–48

Tochner Z, Weshler Z, Rizel S, Fuks Z (1982) Fractionated hemiskeletal irradiation for widespread carcinomatous metastases to bone Int J Radiat Oncol Biol Phys 8: 128 (abstract)

Tong D, Gillick L, Hendrickson FR (1982) The palliation of symptomatic osseous metastases: final results of the study by radiation oncology group. Cancer 50: 893–899

Vargha ZO, Glicksman AS, Boland J (1969) Single-dose radiation therapy in the palliation of metastatic disease. Radiology 93: 1180–1184

Vorobiof DA, Falkson G (1987) Nasally administered buserelin-inducing complete remission of lung metastases in male breast cancer. Cancer 59: 688–689

Zaloznek AJ, Oswald SG, Langin M (1983) Intrapleural tetracycline in malignant pleural effusion. A randomized study. Cancer 51: 752

Zelefsky MJ, Scher HI, Forman JD et al. (1989) Palliative hemiskeletal irradiation for widespread metastatic prostate cancer: a comparison of single-dose and fractionated regiments. Int J Radiat Oncol Biol Phys 17: 1281–1285

37 Carcinomatous Meningitis

B.L. Speiser

A 52-year-old white man received irradiation to the right scapula for an unbiopsied lytic lesion. Within 3 months he became cachectic, with weakness in his lower extremity associated with severe dysphagia. Multiple cranial nerve palsies developed with hydrocephalus, and cerebrospinal fluid (CSF) examination showed many adenocarcinoma cells. Magnetic resonance imaging (MRI) revealed bone marrow replacement in the T11 and L5 vertebrae. He had not walked for the previous 2 weeks, but there was no evidence of epidural cord compression. A large left hilar lung mass was detected.

1. What is the most likely diagnosis?
2. Do you treat carcinomatosis meningitis? How?
3. What is the outcome?
4. What can be expected to improve, symptoms alone or survival?
5. [Include other considerations that would influence your recommendations].

Response

A 52-year-old man with a left hilar mass that was not present 3 months previously, but with presentation of initial metastatic disease to the bone with lytic destruction, both statistically and clinically, would most likely have carcinoma of the lung. Adenocarcinoma, poorly differentiated carcinoma, and large cell carcinoma have slightly higher rates of initial metastasis as compared to squamous cell carcinoma. Small cell carcinoma has the highest rate of initial dissemination, however, it would be unlikely for a patient with a small cell carcinoma to present with a single large lytic lesion and not declare itself in the lung for an additional 3 months. The patient's disease would be consistent with a diffuse meningeal carcinomatosis with more extensive disease in the cauda equina. An MRI scan occasionally can show increase signal intensity along the meningeal lining consistent with meningeal carcinomatosis and occasionally this can also be seen with conventional myelography. In the absence of these radiographic findings, a good neurologic exam will reveal neurologic deficits such as sensory level or levels, decreased proprioception, and/or decreased strength, which will indicate whether spinal cord or spinal root involvement is present. The severe dysphagia that the patient developed is most compatible with a large left hilar mass causing extrinsic compression and possibly direct invasion of the thoracic esophagus. Thus, the most likely diagnosis is adenocarcinoma of the left lung with metastatic disease, both skeletal and meningeal, as evidenced by diffuse meningeal carcinomatosis.

Diffuse meningeal carcinomatosis is a very poor prognostic sign and treatment is most successful when there is a chemotherapeutic regimen available to be used in conjunction with limited radiation. If such a regimen is available, the use of an Ommaya reservoir as a delivery system for chemotherapy is preferred over repeated lumbar taps for intrathecal chemotherapy. For intralumbar administration of chemotherapy, the patient must be kept in a flat or Trendelenburg position for a minimum of 1 h after instillation to ensure adequate flow of the agent to the intraventricular space. The procedure for administration of CSF chemotherapy using the Ommaya reservoir is less demanding, both for the physician and the patient. Once the reservoir is in place, it can be filled by puncturing the skin and reservoir seal with a 23- or 25-gauge scalp vein needle. Most often the area of greatest involvement and the area that is most symptomatic clinically is the cauda equina lumbosacral region. If the patient's Karnofsky status was 30 or below, no treatment would be recommended. If the patient's Karnofsky status was 40–60 inclusive, I would recommend a short course of palliative radiation to the lumbosacral area in an attempt to relieve pain if present and improve neurologic status. With the patient's inability to walk, it is

Burton L. Speiser, MD, St Joseph's Hospital and Medical Center, Department of Radiation Oncology, Phoenix, AZ 85013, USA

assumed that the patient's Karnofsky status is probably no higher than 40. In this case based on the above assumptions, my decision would be to use a short course of palliative radiation to the lumbosacral area, and if clinically indicated, include the T11 vertebral body. If the patient's Karnofsky status was 30 or less and there was no significant pain, I would recommend supportive care. If the patient had leukemia, lymphoma, or breast carcinoma, where effective chemotherapy was still available for that patient, I would advocate the use of the Ommaya reservoir with limited radiation to the lumbosacral area.

The outcome for diffuse meningeal carcinomatosis is quite poor. For patients with a low Karnofsky performance status and the lack of a good systemic and/or central nervous system (CNS) treatment regimen, including chemotherapy, survival tends to be extremely short, usually less than 3 months. However, if the patient has pain as a symptom, this can be expected to improve following radiation. Return of neurologic function, however, is quite dependent on the severity of dysfunction and the time of dysfunction. This patient, who by history had little or no function of the lower extremities for 2 weeks preceding presentation, would have an extremely low probability of neurologic improvement. Based on these assumptions, this patient would require both a Karnofsky status of 40 and other symptoms, such as pain, before advising a course of palliative radiation.

The field would include the T11 vertebral body as opposed to starting just above L1 and extend to S5. The lateral borders would extend to include the transverse processes of the lumbar spine and flare-out to include the sacrum, extending out to the sacroiliac joint. The preferred position for the patient is a prone one. However, many times because of multiple medical and neurologic problems, this is not feasible and most often these patients are treated in a supine fashion over a "tennis racket" with treatment coming through the table. Treatment would be designed as a single posterior field. Calculations are set as the depth to the middle of the spinal cord. If the patient has bulky disease and/or increased symptoms in the sacral distribution, indicating a greater amount of disease, then this area can be boosted to compensate for the greater depth of these structures as compared to the midpoint of the lumbar spinal canal. The overall dose would be 3000 cGy in ten fractions with an optional boost of 600 cGy in two fractions to the sacral region for further disease control. The disadvantage of using a single posterior field is decreased dose homogeneity through a large area, extending from a posterior to anterior direction. However, in this case, the goal of treatment is palliation of meningeal disease where the addition of an anterior field would increase acute morbidity without significant benefit to the patient. The other drawback is the long-term finding of subcutaneous fibrosis with utilizing a single posterior field. This is of very minimal concern for this patient based on the time course for development of subcutaneous fibrosis, which customarily takes 1–2 years before becoming clinically apparent.

38 Adenocarcinoma Metastatic to the Brain

R.H. Sagerman

A 56-year-old black woman had 3 months of tinnitus and then left arm and leg paresthesias. Over the past month, she has experienced short-term memory loss, expressive aphasia, change in mood, and impaired calculation ability. Magnetic resonance imaging (MRI) showed a solitary large frontotemporal tumor with surrounding edema, and a subsequent craniotomy revealed adenocarcinoma. Postoperatively, her moods have been more stable. Chest X-rays and breast examination were normal. An ovarian cyst and a colonic polyp were removed in the past.

1. Would you now irradiate the brain? Why? What is your goal?
2. Is a more extreme work-up indicated at this point?
3. Would you have the histology re-reviewed?
4. [Include other considerations that would influence your recommendation].

Response

Management and clinical judgement in this difficult and tragic situation will be influenced by many social, psychological, economic and medical factors. We will presume that the patient was widowed 8 years earlier, has two adult children, (a working son who is 24 years old and a daughter who is 22 years old and who will earn her Registered Nurse (RN) degree in 6 months) and that she has been self-supporting as a Licensed Practicing Nurse (LPN). Further, we will assume that her past medical history has been relatively benign, that she has no current cardiovascular, gastrointestinal (GI), urological problems or symptoms, and that she underwent natural menopause 4 years previously after an unremarkable menstrual history. We will assume that a large ovarian cyst was discovered at annual gynecological exam, had caused only mild pressure symptoms, was removed transperitoneally without complication, and was reported as a serous cystadenoma. We will also assume that the colonic polyp was removed endoscopically, had caused one episode of rectal bleeding, was pedunculated and 1.5 cm in diameter, and that no malignancy was noted in the specimen.

At the time of consultation with the patient and her children (and it is important to involve this family early), we will confirm that her recent history had been benign, with borderline hypertension (140/95) but with no other organ system complaints, with good appetite and stable weight and that she has never smoked. We will determine that her father died of metastatic colonic carcinoma at age 63 years, her mother of metastatic uterine cancer at age 62 years, and that there has been no other known cancer in her grandparents, brother (52 years) or sisters (61 years and 59 years). Thorough physical examination will be accomplished, documenting her mental state and neurological function, but no primary tumor will be discovered. In particular, no breast mass will be felt, abdominal and pelvic examination will be unremarkable, there will not be any significant peripheral adenopathy, and the lungs will be clear to percussion and auscultation as well as on radiography.

We are, therefore, dealing with a 56-year-old, self-supporting, previously healthy woman with a metastatic adenocarcinoma to the brain from an unknown primary site. I believe that reasonable effort should be expended to try to discover the primary locus, hoping that this will prove to be one of those for which specific, effective treatment may be available. First, the adenocarcinoma should be characterized as completely as possible in hope of suggesting the primary focus. This may involve special staining techniques including immunoperoxidase staging using monoclonal and polyclonal antibodies to characterize enzymes, hormones, normal tissue components, oncofetal antigens, carcinoembryonic antigen, and other proteins. Second, the surgical and pathology records of the ovarian cyst and colonic polyp should be reviewed to insure that these were, indeed, benign lesions. Third, the screening preoperative blood count, urinalysis and biochemical studies should be reviewed, but we will assume they were normal.

Robert H. Sagerman, MD, SUNY Health Science Center, Department of Radiation Oncology, 750 E. Adams Street, Syracuse, NY 13210–2339, USA

Let us presume that the pathologist cannot provide any further help beyond assuring us that this is a garden variety, poorly differentiated, adenocarcinoma and not a lymphoma, melanoma or other unusual tumor. Although we did not discover the primary at physical examination, I would obtain a mammogram as this is relatively simple, cheap and not invasive, and combined modality treatment for disseminated cancer of the breast will sometimes prove very effective. Without suggestive histologic findings, and with an unremarkable physical examination, I would not pursue the thyroid or kidney as likely primaries by performing radionuclide, computed tomographic (CT) or MRI studies. Similarly, I would not do barium studies or colonoscopy to complete a "GI work-up," or pelvic examination under anesthesia with dilation and curettage. Some examiners might conclude that CT is now so readily available and simple that the gut, pancreas, kidneys, and uterus/ovary could be evaluated relatively cheaply, and discover liver metastases, by abdominopelvic scanning, or the lungs by chest scanning, and it is estimated that the primary will be found in 10%–35% of patients, but I would not request these studies for this woman.

Having concluded that we are dealing with metastatic adenocarcinoma to the brain in a previously healthy woman, and not having discovered the primary site, I would consider palliative treatment. We can assume that surgical removal of this "large" lesion with significant temporal lobe involvement is not reasonable by virtue of its size, location and poorly differentiated rather than well-differentiated histology, and would compound the neurological deficits. I would proceed with palliative irradiation, in conjunction with a tapering steroid program, and would normally treat the entire brain, because the vast majority of brain metastases, especially when poorly differentiated, are multifocal, to a dose of 30 Gy delivered in ten fractions. The clinical scenario presented does not require a more rapid program, e.g., 20 Gy in five fractions, 12 Gy in two fractions, and indeed, I would consider an "involved field" boost of 14–20 Gy at 2 Gy/day with the hope of providing longer term tumor control in this previously healthy, self-supporting woman. (This is a program we have employed for many patients with "solitary" brain metastases when the clinical-sociological-psychological situation so warranted, without a discernible risk of or the induction of unusual complications.) I would consider but would not advocate concomitant hyperthermia (too time-consuming), a stereotactic radiotherapy boost (too large a lesion), an implant (invasive second surgical procedure), or nonspecific single agent or multidrug chemotherapy (too toxic?), because none of these treatments have been shown to improve survival of the quality of life to a significant degree.

At diagnosis, only about 5%–10% of cancers are classified as being of unknown primary origin and about 60% are listed as adenocarcinoma. Typically, these patients are elderly and there are multiple metastatic sites. The number, size, and criticality of location determine the presenting signs and symptoms and the liver, lung and bones are most frequently affected. The primary site is discovered during life in about 15%–20% of patients, but is not found even at autopsy in about 25% (Shildt et al. 1983). The lung and pancreas are the most common origins and account for about 40% of cases (Nystrom et al. 1977). The bowel is a frequent site but primary breast, prostate or gynecological cancers rarely present as an "unknown primary."

The median survival for patients with adenocarcinoma of unknown primary site is only 3–4 months, reflecting the poor prognosis in patients with a large tumor burden involving multiple organs. The small subgroup with a better outlook should be searched for so that appropriate treatment can be given and a satisfactory functional state maintained for as long as possible. Accordingly, the light microscopic findings should be followed by immunoperoxidase stains and electron microscopy, but, with the exception of prostate-specific antigen (PSA) staining for prostatic cancer, these are rarely sufficient to pinpoint the primary focus with certainty. Aside from those patients in whom a primary cancer amenable to specific therapy, or with a solitary, well differentiated, small size adenocarcinoma not critically located so that resection with or without adjuvant therapy is feasible, palliative irradiation is usually all that can be done and provides some relief in about two-thirds to three-fourths of patients. The basic concept in this patient is to investigate thoroughly and quickly but not too intrusively and to treat as effectively and rapidly as possible to provide the best qua-lity of life for the longest duration. An honest and thorough discussion with the patient and family is a vital early step and the patient's decision must be respected.

References

Nystrom JS, Weiner JM et al. (1977) Metastatic and histologic presentations in unknown primary cancer. Semin Oncol 4: 53–58

Shildt RA, Kennedy PS et al. (1983) Management of patients with metastatic adenocarcinoma of unknown origin: a Southwest Oncology Group study. Cancer Treat Rep 67: 77–79

39 Craniopharyngioma

J.R. CASSADY

During follow-up examination after a surgical procedure to correct bilateral ureteropelvic junction strictures, an exotropic and nonreactive pupil was found in this 3-year-old boy. Optic atrophy was found in both eyes, but visual acuity was good. A large cystic craniopharyngioma with extension under the temporal lobe was successfully removed, except for the inferior portion of the cystic capsule. Within the next 6 months, the cystic portion of the craniopharyngioma reformed and necessitated aspiration twice. When seen by the radiation oncologist, the patient was practically blind.

1. Should this patient have been irradiated immediately postoperatively?
2. What are the risks of irradiating a "young" brain?
3. Would a biopsy plus radiations alone have resulted in a better outcome?
4. Are craniopharyngiomas radiosensitive? Should they ever be irradiated without tissue confirmation?
5. [Include other considerations that would influence your recommendation].

Response

Conservative surgery (cyst aspiration, biopsy or conservative subtotal removal) combined with three-field or rotational megavoltage irradiation has consistently been demonstrated to result in both optimum long-term tumor control and equivalent or superior functional status for patients with craniopharyngioma (FISCHER et al. 1985, 1990; WEISS et al. 1989; RICHMOND et al. 1980). Attempts at "total" tumor removal, including recent reports utilizing modern, microsurgical techniques consistently demonstrate a substantial incidence of incomplete tumor removal or recurrence following apparent "total" removal (WEISS et al. 1989; KATZ 1980; MANAKA et al. 1985). In addition, a virtually uniform need for multiple pituitary hormone replacement and postoperative diabetes insipidus as well as the possibility of hypothalamic injury, frontal lobe dysfunction, intellectual disturbances (including intelligence quotient, IQ, deficits), visual abnormalities and a significant incidence of vascular accidents and stroke often result from these aggressive attempts (FISCHER et al. 1990; WEISS et al. 1989; KATZ 1980; GALATZER et al. 1981).

Most patients with craniopharyngioma are more than 7 years of age when first seen (MANAKA et al. 1985). In a recent large series reported from Japan, nearly 58% of 125 patients were more than 14 years of age when first seen. Even if one limits analysis to children less than 16 years of age, presentation before the age of 5 years is distinctly uncommon, and diagnosis at age 3 years as with the child under discussion is fortunately quite rare.

Treatment of the immature brain with high doses of irradiation may produce a variety of undesirable sequelae. Use of moderate or high doses (3500–5500 cGy) of irradiation may produce a vascular developmental arrest in which arteries and arterioles in the treatment field fail to enlarge as the child grows older with resultant arterial insufficiency and a myoma-like syndrome or stroke. In addition, a variety of other neurologic sequelae may result including pituitary hormone deficits (growth hormone production is most sensitive), diabetes insipidus, intellectual disturbances or learning disabilities. These sequelae are dose and volume-dependant and are also influenced by concurrent or postirradiation chemotherapy especially when methotrexate is used concurrent with or following irradiation. In the child under discussion, arterial developmental abnormalities, deficits in pituitary hormone secretion, diabetes insipidus, mild-to-moderate intellectual deficits and learning disabilities are all possible sequelae of treatment (MEADOWS et al. 1981; MECHANICK et al. 1986; MARKS and WONG 1985; SHALET et al. 1990).

J. Robert Cassady, MD, University of Arizona Health Sciences Center, Department of Radiation Oncology, 1501 North Campbell Avenue, Tucson, AZ 85724, USA

Because of these potential adverse effects and because development, maturation, and myelinization of the nervous system continues until age 5 years or beyond, it has become common practice in the treatment of both malignant and benign brain tumors in childhood to attempt to delay irradiation until age 4 or 5 years through the use of surgery and where appropriate, chemotherapy. However, this approach is only warranted when frequent and careful observation is possible and, should any neurologic worsening or objective tumor growth occur, treatment with irradiation should take place.

The initial approach in this child of conservative subtotal removal and observation without irradiation therefore seems reasonable considering the child's young age. However, subsequent management was not optimal and resulted in considerable unnecessary neurologic disability. Following initial surgery, we would have recommended careful observation combined with frequent imaging and visual field studies. Despite inclusion in a text discussing palliative approaches, this child should at all times be considered a candidate for cure and subsequent long-term survival. Following initial evidence of tumor regrowth, rather than simple cyst aspiration, we would have favored combined cyst aspiration with a short course or multiagent, cytotoxic chemotherapy. FISCHER et al. (1990) report an "impressive reduction" in tumor following a brief course of nitrogen mustard, Oncovin (vincristine), procarbazine, and prednisone (MOPP) chemotherapy and BREMER et al. (1984) report similar regression following vincristine, 1,3-bis-(2-chlorethyl)-1-nitroso-urea (BCNU) and procarbazine. Instillation of bleomycin in the cyst cavity has resulted in variable results (TAKAHAYASHI et al. 1985). Although intracyst instillation of yttrium-90 has also been recommended, we would not favor this in the child under discussion, as this approach is not likely to result in permanent tumor control and may considerably compromise external beam treatment options in the future. Similarly, stereotaxic radiosurgery has been utilized in this setting in some patients, however, the long-term functional results are unknown and optimal technical treatment factors (such as total dose or field size) are unclear and no convincing long-term tumor control results have been published.

We would not favor a chemotherapy approach requiring more than three full cycles of MOPP or similar chemotherapy in order to minimize potential long-term toxicity such as sterility and leukemia. As craniopharyngioma results from growth or an embryonic remnant of Rathke's pouch, it is not surprising that rapid tumor recurrence was noted in this child. Collins (1955) has described a relationship between age at presentation of an embryonal tumor (Wilm's) and time to recurrence which suggests that embryonal tumors that present at a young age are likely, if not fully controlled, to recur in a relatively short time (age at presentation plus 9 months). This relationship has been confirmed in medulloblastoma and neuroblastoma, and it is therefore not surprising that rapid clinical reappearance of tumor developed in this unusually young child with craniopharyngioma who had known residual tumor.

Should cytotoxic chemotherapy not result in tumor response or, following response from the course of chemotherapeutic treatment recommended, tumor regrowth develop, we would then favor implementing a course of external beam radiotherapy immediately.

We are unaware of any in vitro data which addresses the question regarding radiosensitivity of craniopharyngioma. However, clinical control of tumor regularly accompanies fractionated irradiation courses of more than 5000–54000 cGy provided that adequate treatment volumes have been treated (FISCHER et al. 1985, 1990; MANAKA et al. 1985). We feel that one reason that irradiation, following one or more surgical recurrences of craniopharyngioma, results in somewhat lower overall control rates is due to tumor contamination of the surgical bed. Although infrequent, recurrences in these patients are, on occasion, noted to be in unusual sites such as in the anterior cranial fossa in a subfrontal location or in a subtemporal or even clival location. Therefore, when patients with one or more postsurgical recurrences are treated, relatively generous fields should be used.

We do not feel that radiation doses should be "adjusted" for patient age. Therefore, a minimum dose of 5000 cGy should be used and most series reporting high long-term control rates use a minimum dose of 5400–5500 cGy utilizing an arc-rotation or three-field approach. As a technical point, the exit-component of either an arc-rotation or vertex field should be directed to avoid the thyroid gland in any pediatric or young adult patient. Alternatively, fractionated external beam treatment to 45 Gy followed by a radiosurgical "boost" may be an alternative with less late toxicity and equal control probability. However, no long-term control or complication data exist for this approach. Finally, fractionated daily radiosurgery potentially offers an optimal outcome as a future possibility.

Results of radiation treatment are generally optimal when surgery has been limited to cyst aspiration or biopsy only. We feel that cyst aspiration which reveals typical "crankcase fluid" filled with cholesterol crystals is sufficient documentation of a craniopharyngioma and, when obtained, additional tissue documentation is not required prior to irradiation. This approach minimizes the risk of surgical morbidity, eliminates the risk of subtle frontal lobe dysfunctions which have been described by Cavazutti following more extensive surgery and leads to excellent long-term results (CAVAZZUTI et al. 1983; CLOPPER et al. 1983). With this approach, one or more cyst aspirations are often needed during or following irradiation in this slowly responding tumor prior to clinical tumor control.

Functional results in most childhood patients treated with conservative surgery and irradiation are excellent (FISCHER et al. 1985, 1990; WEISS et al. 1989). Although development of a radiation associated tumor is a possibility, this has fortunately been a rare occurrence (FISCHER et al. 1990).

It is likely that initial biopsy followed by irradiation would have led to a better visual functional outcome in the child under discussion, however, more rapid institution of irradiation following recurrence (progression) would likely have achieved this same outcome and hopefully would have permitted some similarly young children to avoid the potential developmental toxicities of irradiation by delaying radiation treatment.

References

Bremer AM, Nguyen TQ, Balsys R (1984) Therapeutic benefits of combination chemotherapy with vincristine, BCNU and procarbazine on recurrent craniopharyngiomas: a case report. J Neurooncol 2: 47–51

Cavazzuti V, Fischer EG, Welch K et al (1983) Neurological and psycho physiological sequelae following different treatments of craniopharyngiomas in children. J Neurosurg 59: 409–417

Clopper RR, Meyer WL III, Udrahelyi GB et al. (1983) Postsurgical IQ and behavioral data on twenty patients with a history of childhood craniopharyngiomas. Psychoneuroendocrinology, 2: 365–372

Collins VP (1955) Wilm's tumor: its behavior and prognosis. J La State Med Soc 197: 474–480

Fischer EG, Welch K, Belli JA et al. (1985) Treatment of craniopharyngiomas in children. J Neurosurg 62: 496 – 501

Fischer EG, Welch K, Shillito J, Winston KR, Tarbell NJ (1990) Craniopharyngiomas in children: long-term effects of conservative surgical procedures combined with radiation therapy. J Neurosurg 73: 534–540

Galatzer A, Nofar E, BenHalachini N et al. (1981) Intellectual and psychosocial functions of children, adolescents and young adults before and after operation for craniopharyngiomas. Child Care Health Dev 7: 307–316

Katz EL (1980) Late results of radical excision of craniopharyngiomas in children. J Neurosurg 42: 86–90

Manaka S, Teramoto A, Takakura K (1985) The efficacy of radiotherapy for craniopharyngiomas. J Neurosurg 62: 648–656

Marks J, Wong J (1985) The risk of cerebral radionecrosis in relation to dose, time and fractionation. Prog Exp Tumor Res 29: 210–218

Meadows AT, Gordon J, Massari DJ et al. (1981) Declines in IQ scores and cognitive dysfunctions in children with acute lymphoblastic leukemia treated with cranial radiation. Lancet 2: 1015–1018

Mechanick JI, Hochberg FH, LaRocque A (1986) Whole brain irradiation. J Neurosurg 65: 490–494

Richmond IL, Wara WM, Wilson CG (1980) Role of radiation therapy in the management of craniopharyngiomas in children. Neurosurg 6: 513–517

Shalet SM, OgilvyStuart AL, Crowne EC, Clayton PE (1990) Indications for human growth hormone treatment of radiation-induced growth hormone deficiency. In: Green DM, DAngio CJ (eds) Late effects of treatment for childhood cancer. Wiley-Liss, New York, pp 71–79

Takahayashi H, Nakazawa S, Shimura T (1985) Evaluation of postoperative intratumeral injection of bleomycin for craniopharyngiomas in children. J Neurosurg 62: 120 – 127

Weiss M, Sutton L, Marcial V et al. (1989) The role of radiation therapy in the management of childhood craniopharyngiomas. Int J Radiat Oncol Biol Phys 17: 1313–1321

40 Metastatic Cancer Involving the Eye

L.W. Brady, J.A. Shields, C.L. Shields, J.C. Hernandez, and B. Micaily

Ten years ago this 52-year-old woman had a stage II adenocarcinoma of the left breast (estrogen receptor/progesterone receptor – ER/PR – positive) managed by a modified mastectomy and 1 year of adjuvant chemotherapy. Her present complaint is decreasing vision in her left eye. Visual acuity is 20/400 and ultrasound shows a mass in the choroid which corresponds to an 8-disk diameter mass in the inferior temporal portion of the fundus.

1. What would you recommend?
2. Systemic management?
3. Dose-time relationship?
4. Treatment of the contralateral eye?
5. How would you recommend change if the patient had associated lung and symptomatic brain metastasis?
6. What is the error in treating without a histologic diagnosis?
7. [Include other considerations that would influence your recommendation].

Response

The critical issue in managing the patient outlined above is the determination of the general disease state within the patient. The onset of decreasing vision in the left eye with a mass demonstrated in the choroid by ultrasound indicates the potential diagnosis of metastatic carcinoma to the choroid of the eye. The location of the mass in the inferior temporal portion of the fundus corresponding to a size of 8 disk diameters is compatible with the diagnosis. However, with the interval of 10 years from the original diagnosis to the development of the metastatic lesion of the eye indicates that other potential diagnoses should be considered. Therefore, a fine needle aspirate biopsy would be appropriate to establish the diagnosis.

L.W. Brady, MD, J. C. Hernandez, MD, B. Micaily, MD
Hahnemann University, Department of Radiation Oncology, Philadelphia, PA, USA
J.A. Shields, MD, C.L. Shields, MD, Wills Eye Hospital, Ocular Oncology Service, Philadelphia, PA, USA

Table 1. Location of primary malignancy in 300 patients with metastatic tumors to the intraocular structures (From Green 1986, and Bullock and Yanes 1980)

Primary location	Number	Percentage[a]
Breast	162	54
Lung	68	23
Undetermined	24	8
Alimentary tract	22	7
Skin (melanoma)	11	4
Kidney	5	2
Thyroid	4	1
Prostate	2	1
Larynx	2	1

[a] Figures do not add up to 100% because of rounding

In the decision-making process in the management of this tumor being metastatic to the choroid of the eye is the decision as to whether it exists as a single metastatic lesion or is a part of multiple metastatic lesions. Therefore, it is appropriate to proceed to do an adequate appropriate work-up to define the true extent of the disease process. Therefore, the decision with regards to systemic disease is very important and particularly whether the systemic disease is under control, absent or uncontrolled. The metastatic lesion of the eye occurring 10 years after the original diagnosis and in the absence of systemic disease would represent a autochronous metastatic lesion.

The decision-making process in the management is set forth in Table 1 based on whether it is a single metastasis or whether it is a part of multiple metastatic lesions (Figs. 1, 2). The final decision for treatment would depend upon where the patient falls in the decision tree. In the situation of a single metastasis with no systemic disease, definitive treatment to the eye is warranted. However, a single metastasis involving the choroid of the eye with systemic disease would warrant palliative radiotherapy to the metastatic lesion of the eye and multiple adjuvant, systemic chemotherapy. On the other hand, if the lesion represents one of multiple lesions but limited

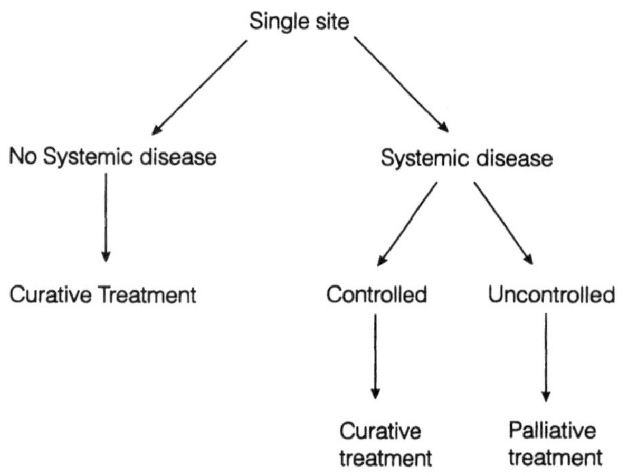

Fig. 1. Metastatic tumors to the eye: single site

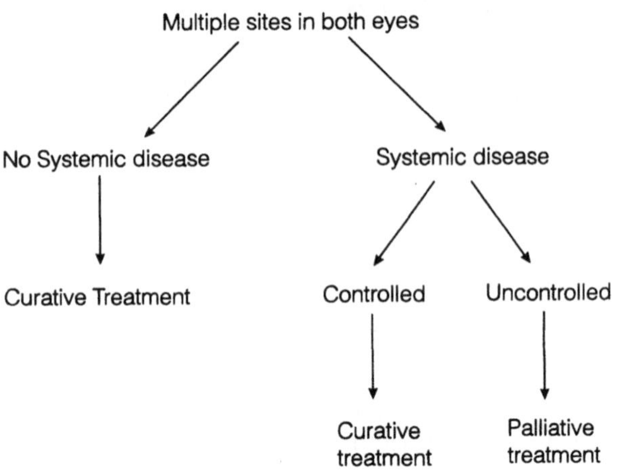

Fig. 2. Metastatic tumors to the eye: multiple sites

to the eye with no systemic disease definitive treatment would still be warranted, but on the other hand with active systemic disease, palliative treatment to the eye would be warranted along with adjuvant systemic chemotherapy.

Neoplasms that metastasize to the ocular structures constitute a group of tumors that are of major importance to oncologists, ophthalmologists and other specialists (FERRY and FONT 1974; JENSEN 1975; SHIELDS et al. 1990, 1991). The ophthalmologist plays a major role in the diagnosis and follow-up of these patients. An intraocular metastatic tumor is a malignant neoplasm that has spread via hematogenous dissemination to the uveal tract but also may involve the retina, the optic disk or other structures within the eye. From a historical point of view metastatic cancer to the eye represents a relatively rare disease. In 1944, CORDES stated that few ophthalmologists had seen more than one case. However by 1950 the incidence had increased considerably and with the advent of more effective systemically administered chemotherapy agents and more effective local and regional treatment programs, metastatic lesions to the eye are being seen more commonly now than ever before (GREEAR 1950; SPAETH 1951; DUKEELDER and PERKINS 1966; ALBERT et al. 1967; GOTFREDSEN 1944; VON GUTHBERT et al. 1965; BLACK and GARTNER 1971; GILLET 1971; FERRY and FONT 1974; FRANCOIS et al. 1976). It has been estimated in 1992 that metastatic cancer to the uvea is the most common form of intraocular malignancy. However, many cases are never diagnosed because the metastasis occurs in a patient who is extremely ill or in the terminal state of the illness where ocular examination is not routinely performed. It is frequent for patients to appear physically well and to have ocular metastasis.

The total incidence of ocular metastasis in all patients dying from all types of carcinoma is about 4%. The estimate in 1983 was for 22 000 patients who would have metastatic cancer to the eye (NELSON et al. 1983). This is a far greater incidence than that of primary uveal melanomas. It has been suggested that the apparent increased incidence of metastatic intraocular tumors is due to longer survival of patients with a variety of cancers as well as improved clinical detection of metastatic tumors by ophthalmologists and other specialists (GILLET 1971; STEPHENS and SHIELDS 1979).

In the joint program between Wills Eye Hospital Oncology Service and the Department of Radiation Oncology at Hahnemann University, more than 300 consecutive patients with metastatic tumors to the uvea were seen in the period from 1974 to 1989 (SHAKIN et al., manuscript in preparation). Of these metastatic lesions, 95% occurred in white patients, 4% in black patients and 1% in Hispanic patients.

The majority of intraocular metastases are from carcinomas of various sites, with it being extremely rare for sarcomas to metastasize to the uvea (FERRY and FONT 1974). Cutaneous malignant melanoma can metastasize to the uvea particularly when the patient has widespread disseminated disease (DEBUSTROS et al. 1985; FERRY 1972). Table 1 indicates the location of the primary malignancy among the 300 patients with metastatic tumors to intraocular structures (SHAKIN et al., manuscript in preparation; GREEN 1986).

Among the reported series, breast cancer represents the greatest majority of intraocular metastatic lesions. The majority of affected patients have a history of breast cancer, but occasionally the intraocular metastasis represents the first clinical manifestation of systemic disease (Shakin et al., manuscript in preparation; Bullock and Yanes 1980; Lakhanpal et al. 1982; Mew and Young 1982; Reynard and Font 1983).

Metastatic lung cancer to the uvea sometimes occurs before the primary tumor is recognized. In general, lung cancer constitutes 23% of the intraocular metastasis (Crawford and Reese 1969; Jarrett et al. 1970; Klein et al. 1977; Kreiger et al. 1969; Levine and Williamson 1970; Young et al. 1979). The other sites are alimentary tract, skin and other organs (Karnad 1986; Kennedy et al. 1958; Michelson et al. 1975; Mullaney 1970; Rootman and Butler 1982). The majority of metastatic lesions to the uvea occur in women, representing an incidence of 70% where the most common primary source was breast cancer. In men lung cancer was the primary tumor in 44% of the cases (Green 1986; Bullock and Yanes 1980).

One of the most important diagnostic aspects in the evaluation of a patient with a suspected intraocular metastatic tumor is the history of a prior primary malignancy established in the past. The clinical diagnosis of metastatic uveal tumor is often greatly facilitated in patients with a positive history, whereas the diagnosis may be more difficult in patients with a negative history. In the Wills eye series, 27% of patients who had intraocular metastases had no history of a primary malignancy when they were first seen by the ophthalmologist. A history of primary breast cancer was present in 92% of the patients with uveal metastases. In the remaining cases, the primary tumor often was diagnosed by breast examination or mammographic examination shortly after the ocular lesion was detected.

The vast majority of intraocular metastases are found in the uvea but metastatic lesions can occur to the retina, the vitreous and the optic disk although much less common. Metastatic lesions are more likely to occur bilaterally than are primary uveal melanomas. This emphasizes the need for careful ophthalmologic examination of both eyes (Shakin et al., manuscript in preparation).

Another feature of metastatic tumors to the uvea is their tendency to be multifocal in one or both eyes. Multifocal metastases occurred in 32% of the eyes with metastases from breast carcinoma and in 22% from lung cancers (Shakin et al., manuscript in preparation). Multiple foci are not surprising since the terminal branches of the ciliary arteries supply the choriocapillaries in a segmental pattern.

The clinical features of metastatic tumors to the intraocular structures vary with the location of the tumor in the eye (Shields et al. 1991). A patient with a metastatic tumor to the choroid may be asymptomatic or may experience painless blurred vision. In rare instances, pain caused by secondary glaucoma may be the initial manifestation. Ophthalmologic examination of a choroidal metastasis characteristically reveals a homogenous, creamy yellow placoid lesion in the posterior choroid. Tumors that are slightly more elevated frequently produce a serous detachment of the fovea and alterations in the retinal pigment epithelium. The retinal pigment epithelium changes can be rather marked appearing as well-delineated clumps of golden-brown pigment on the surface of the tumor. In some instances, the tumor may appear multinodular. In contrast to carcinomas, metastatic melanomas to the choroid are usually mild to moderately pigmented. In some instances, a metastatic choroid tumor can be highly elevated and have a dome shape similar to a primary amelanotic melanoma. Secondary proliferation and migration of the retinal pigment epithelium on the surface of the tumor may further suggest the diagnosis of melanoma. In such instances, an intensive clinical evaluation may be necessary to establish the diagnosis. Serous detachment of the sensory retina is associated with a metastatic choroidal tumor in about 75% of cases (Shakin et al., manuscript in preparation). In some instances, it involves only the fovea adjacent to the tumor, whereas in other cases it may bullous. When the detachment is extensive, dramatic shifting of the subretinal fluid can be demonstrated with movements of the patient's head. Rarely, atypical cases of choroidal metastases that break through Bruch's membrane and assume a mushroom shape. However, this finding is much more common with primary uveal melanomas. Metastatic tumors to the choroid, particularly those from a lung primary, can occasionally produce a peripheral choroidal detachment and simulate a uveal effusion syndrome. When they extend anteriorly into the ciliary region, there may be an associated tortuous episcleral blood vessel similar to that seen in some eyes with primary melanoma. The reactive vascularity may be so severe that the diagnosis of scleritis is made (Yeo et al. 1983).

There are a number of conditions that can clinically simulate a metastatic cancer to the choroid and should be considered in the differential diagnosis.

These include amelanotic nevus, amelanotic melanoma, choroidal hemangioma, posterior scleritis, choroidal osteoma, retinitis, choroiditis, rhegmatogenous retinal detachment, Harada's disease, uveal effusion syndrome, and central serous chorioretinopathy. A detailed history is often very helpful in making the differentiation but the ophthalmoscopic differences are also very important.

Ciliary body metastases are often difficult to detect, since they may clinically masquerade as a chronic uveitis or secondary glaucoma. They may occur as the initial manifestation of rare occult primary neoplasms, such as carcinoma of the common bile duct and carcinoid tumor of the thymus (LIEB et al. 1990).

Another problem is the potential for iris metastasis (FERRY and FONT 1975). These are often asymptomatic or with only mild visual symptoms in the involved eye. However, pain caused by severe inflammation or secondary glaucoma may be the presenting manifestation in some instances (LIEB et al. 1990; WOOG et al., 1984).

Metastatic tumors of the retina are extremely rare, and only a small number of cases have been reported (YOUNG et al. 1979; KENNEDY et al. 1958; LETSON and DAVIDORF 1982). In contrast to choroidal metastasis, retinal metastases are less cohesive and may seed tumor cells into the vitreous. They sometimes resemble a retinitis more closely than they resemble a true tumor.

Metastatic tumors may also develop in the optic papilla of secondary to tumor emboli in the small vessels of the disk or by direct extension from the adjacent choroidal tumor (LIEB et al. 1990; WOOG et al. 1984).

From the diagnostic point of view, a number of ancillary ophthalmic procedures may aid in the diagnosis of metastatic tumors. These include not only the systemic evaluation but fluorescein angiography, ultrasonography, computed tomography (CT), magnetic resonance imaging (MRI), radioactive phosphorus (32P) test, needle aspirate biopsy or wedge biopsy.

Therefore, in every patient presenting with a metastatic lesion to the choroid must have a systemic evaluation to identify the true state of the disease process. This would include not only a careful history and physical examination but appropriate mammographic examinations, chest X-rays, bone scans, CT scans of the abdomen and pelvis, other studies directed to other organ sites as well as proper and appropriate studies of the tumor itself including the ophthalmologic studies.

In some instances where the diagnosis is difficult, a fine needle aspirate biopsy can be used to establish the diagnosis. This technique is straightforward for lesions in the iris but requires greater expertise for lesions located in the posterior segment of the eye. It can be done safely and without significant complications allowing for appropriate and proper cytologic examination of the specimen removed. The risk related to the fine needle aspiration biopsy is negligible. When the needle aspiration does not yield enough cells to establish a definitive diagnosis of metastatic carcinoma to the ciliary body or choroid, a wedge biopsy via a scleral flap can be done. This method obtains more tissue allowing the pathologist to be more specific in the diagnosis but it does carry with it more risk of complication.

The preferred treatment for intraocular metastasis depends upon the degree of activity in the tumor, the patient's symptoms, the degree of control obtainable with chemotherapy, the location and extent of the tumor and the site of the primary tumor. It may involve simple observation, radiotherapy or surgical resection. Observation is pursued when the tumor is not active and asymptomatic.

It has been reported that chemotherapy systemically administered may benefit positively the response of the tumor. However, the single most important treatment program is the use of radiotherapy in the management of the metastasis. The entire posterior segment of the globe is irradiated using a temporal and/or anteromedial field with 30–40 Gy being delivered in fractionated radiotherapy over a 4-week period of time. In those patients where the metastasis involving the eye is the only evidence of disease, a more aggressive program of radiotherapy would be pursued delivering 50–60 Gy in 5.5–6 weeks depending upon the histologic character of the tumor. In general, the program pursued in the Wills Eye Hospital/Hahnemann University cooperative effort uses field setups such as illustrated in Fig. 3.

Following radiotherapy, choroidal metastasis shows a decreasing thickness, disappearance of the secondary retinal detachment, and proliferation of the overlying retinal pigment epithelium. The visual acuity often shows a dramatic improvement in successfully treated patients. In some instances brachytherapy may be used to treat the tumor using a radioactive episcleral plaque. In general, this has been limited to metastases to the uvea where the dose to the apex of the tumor is 35 Gy. The method works well and gives rise to excellent responses and excellent control. Enucleation or local surgical excision of

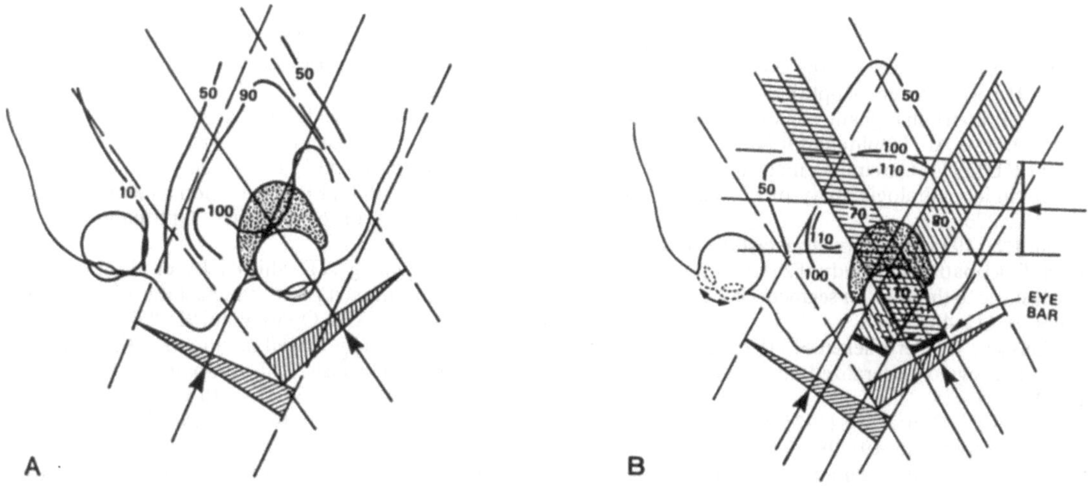

Fig. 3. A Isodose distribution using the isocentric technique for a unilateral treatment volume (*stippled area*). *Numbers* indicate percentages of the absorbed dose at the isocenter. Two wedged oblique fields are used to optimize the 90% isodose contour to the treatment volume. **B** At the level of the lens, an eye bar is inserted in both oblique fields with the patient looking at the eye bar for each oblique treatment field

a metastatic tumor may be justified because of size or intractable pain.

Summary

Metastatic tumors to the eye are now recognized to be the most common type of intraocular malignancy although many cases are never diagnosed clinically. The choroid is the most common site of involvement and metastases to the ciliary body, iris, retina, and optic nerve are considerably less common. About 27% of patients who are seen with ocular metastases have no history of prior malignancy.

The tumors that most commonly metastasize to the eye originate from breast carcinoma in women and from lung cancer in men. Less commonly, ocular metastases occur from the alimentary tract, thyroid, kidney, pancreas and other organs. Malignant melanomas can metastasize to the uvea from a cutaneous primary site or from a primary uveal site in the opposite eye. Although most metastatic tumors have a rather typical clinical appearance with ophthalmoscopy or slit lamp biomicroscopy, occasionally they may be confused with other intraocular tumor or inflammatory processes. Studies such as fluorescein angiography, ultrasonography, CT, MRI, may provide diagnostic information. Occasionally, a fine needle biopsy or a wedge biopsy may be necessary to establish the diagnosis firmly.

The single most important treatment program directed toward management is radiation therapy. It offers the opportunity for local control in a high percentage of the patients treated and with preservation of vision. The decision with regards to radiation dose to be delivered is dependent upon the presence or absence of systemic disease and whether the patient is treated for palliation or cure. In the absence of systemic disease with a single lesion in the eye, the patient should always be given the option for treatment for cure.

References

Albert DM, Rubenstein RA, Scheie HG (1967) Tumor metastasis to the eye. Part 1: incidence in 213 adult patients with generalized malignancy. Am J Ophthalmol 63: 723–776

Bloch RS, Gartner S (1971) The incidence of ocular metastatic carcinoma. Arch Ophthalmol 85: 673–675

Bullock JD, Yanes B (1980) Ophthalmic manifestations of metastatic breast cancer. Ophthalmology 87: 961–973

Cordes FC (1944) Bilateral metastatic carcinoma of the choroid with X-ray therapy to one eye: report of a case. Am J Ophthalmol 27: 1355–1370

Crawford JB, Reese GA (1969) Rapid loss of vision: initial manifestation of bronchogenic carcinoma (a clinicopathologic case report). Trans Am Acad Ophthalmol Otolaryngol 73: 964–968

deBustros S, Augsburger JJ, Shields JA et al. (1985) Intraocular metastases from cutaneous malignant melanoma. Arch Ophthalmol 103: 937–940

DukeElder S, Perkins ES (1966) Diseases of the uveal tract. In: DukeElder S (ed) Diseases of the uveal tract. Mosby, St. Louis, pp 919–937 (System of ophthalmology vol 9.)

Ferry AP (1972) Primary malignant melanoma of the skin metastatic to the eye. Am J Ophthalmol 74: 12–19

Ferry AP, Font RL (1974) Carcinoma metastatic to the eye and orbit: a clinicopathologic study of 227 cases. Arch Ophthalmol 92: 276–286

Ferry AP, Font RL (1975) Carcinoma metastatic to the eye and orbit: a clinicopathologic study of 26 patients with carcinoma metastatic to the anterior segment of the eye. Arch Ophthalmol 29: 472–482

Francois J, Hanssens H, Verbraeken H (1976) Intraocular metastasis as first sign of generalized carcinomatosis. Ann Ophthalmol 8: 405–419

Gallie BL, Graham JE, Hunter WS (1975) Optic nerve head metastasis. Arch Ophthalmol 93: 983–986

Gillet RB (1971) Metastatic carcinoma of the choroid. Tex Med 67: 72–75

Gotfredsen E (1944) On the frequency of secondary carcinomas in the choroid. Acta Ophthalmol 22: 394–400

Greear JN Jr (1950) Metastatic carcinoma of the eye. Am J Ophthalmol 33: 10157–1025

Green WR (1986) The uveal tract. In: Spencer WH, Font RL, Green WR et al. (eds) Ophthalmic pathology: an atlas and textbook. Saunders, Philadelphia, pp1645–1655

Jarrett WH Jr, Green WR, Berlin AJ Jr et al. (1970) Retinal detachment as the initial manifestation of carcinoma of the lung. Trans Am Acad Ophthalmol Otolaryngol 74: 52–58

Jensen OA (1975) Metastatic tumors of the eye and orbit: a histopathological analysis of a Danish series. Acta Pathol Microbiol Immunol Scand 212 [Suppl]: 201–214

Karnad A, Poskit TR, Lines LG et al. (1986) Simultaneous bilateral ocular metastases from a gastric carcinoma. Ann Ophthalmol 18: 188–190

Kennedy RJ, Rummel WD, McCarthy JL et al. (1958) Metastatic carcinoma of the retina. Arch Ophthalmol 60: 1–18

Klein R, Nicholson DH, Luxenberg MN (1977) Retinal metastasis from squamous cell carcinoma of the lung. Am J Ophthalmol 83: 358–361

Kreiger AE, Meyer D, Smith TR et al. (1969) Metastatic carcinoma to the choroid with choroidal detachment: a case presenting as uveal effusion. Arch Ophthalmol 82: 209–213

Lakhanpal V, Dardsh J, Schocket S et al. (1982) Bilateral choroidal metastases from male breast carcinoma. Ann Ophthalmol 14: 982–984

Letson AD, Davidorf FH (1982) Bilateral retinal metastases from cutaneous melanoma. Arch Ophthalmol 100: 605–607

Levine RA, Williamson DE (1970) Metastatic carcinoma simulating a postoperative endophthalmitis. Arch Ophthalmol 83: 59–61

Lieb WE, Shields JA, Shields CL et al. (1990) Mucinous adenocarcinoma metastatic to the iris, ciliary body, and choroid. Br J Ophthalmol 74: 373–376

Mew L, Young SE (1982) Breast carcinoma metastatic to the choroid: analysis of 67 patients. Ophthalmology 89: 147–151

Michelson JB, Felberg NT, Shields JA et al. (1975) Carcinoembryonic antigen positive metastatic adenocarcinoma of the choroid. Arch Ophthalmol 93: 794–796

Mullaney J (1970) Squamous cell carcinoma of the esophagus with choroidal metastasis. Br J Ophthalmol 544: 281–283

Nelson CC, Hertzberg BS, Klintworth GK (1983) A histopathologic study of 716 unselected eyes in patients with cancer at the time of death. Am J Ophthalmol 95: 788–793

Norton HJ (1959) Adenocarcinoma metastatic to the distal nerve and optic disc. Am J Ophthalmol 47: 195–199

Reynard M, Font RL (1983) Two cases of uveal metastases from breast carcinoma in men. Am J Ophthalmol 95: 208–215

Rootman J, Butler D (1982) Consecutive bilateral ocular metastases from an asymptomatic adenocarcinoma of the cardia. Can J Ophthalmol 17: 79–81

Shakin EP, Shields JA, Shields CL. (in preparation) Metastatic cancer to the uvea: a survey of 300 cases.

Shields JA, Shakin EP, Shields CL (1990) Neoplasms metastatic to the eye and adnexa. In: Gold DH, Weingeist TA (eds) The eye in systemic disease. Lippincott, Philadelphia

Shields JA, Char DH, Foulds WS et al. (1991): Intraocular metastatic tumors. In: Singerman LJ, Jampol LM (eds) Retinal and choroidal manifestations of systemic disease.

Spaeth EB (1951) Ocular tumors: a study of incidence of the various types and their mortality rates. Arch Ophthalmol 46: 421–423

Stephens RF, Shields JA (1979) Diagnosis and management of cancer metastatic to the uvea: a study of 70 cases. Ophthalmology 86: 1336–1349

Von Guthbert H, Janisch W, Rossbach K (1965) Über die Häufigkeit der Augenmetastasen. Munch Med Wochenschr 10 107: 939–941

Woog JJ, Chess J, Albert DM et al. (1984) Metastatic carcinoma of the iris simulating iridocyclitis. Br J Ophthalmol 68: 167–173

Yeo JH, Jakobiec FA, Iwamoto T et al. (1983) Metastatic carcinoma masquerading as scleritis. Ophthalmology 90: 184–194

Young SE, Cruciger M, Lukeman J (1979) Metastatic carcinoma to the retina: a case report. Ophthalmology 86: 1350–1354

List of Contributors

BERNARD S. ARON, MD
University of Cincinnati Medical Center
Department of Radiation Oncology
Cincinnati, OH 45 267–0757
USA

SUCHA O. ASBELL, MD
Department of Radiation Oncology
Albert Einstein Medical Center
5501 Old York Road
Philadelphia, PA 19141–3096
USA

J.A. BATTLE, MD
Department of Radiation Oncology
Medical College of Ohio
P.O. Box 1008
Toledo, OH 43699–0008
USA

JOHN BEDWINEK, MD
Radiation Therapy Department
St. John's Mercy Medical Center
615 S. New Ballas Road
St. Louis, MO 63141
USA

WYMAN A. BETHUNE, MD
Department of Radiation Oncology
University Hospital Health Science Center
Suny at Stony Brook
Stony Brook, NY 11794–7028
USA

LUTHER W. BRADY, MD
Professor and chairman
Department of Radiation Oncology and Nuclear Medicine
Hahnemann University
230 N. Broad St., M.S. 200
Philadelphia, PA 19102
USA

THEODORE J. BRICKNER, JR, MD
Department of Radiation Oncology
Natalie Warren Bryant Cancer Center
St. Francis Hospital
6161 South Yale Avenue
Tulsa, OK 74136
USA

THOMAS A. BUCHHOLZ, MD
Department of Radiation Oncology
University of Washington, Medical Center RC-08
1959 N. E. Pacific
Seattle, WA 98195
USA

J. ROBERT CASSADY, MD
Department of Radiation Oncology
University of Arizona
Health Sciences Center
1501 North Campbell Avenue
Tucson, AZ 85724
USA

JOSEPH R. CASTRO, MD
Director, Radiation Oncology
Lawrence Berkeley Laboratory
1 Cyclotron Road
Berkeley, CA 94720
USA

CHAHIN M. CHAHBAZIAN, MD
Radiation Oncology
Medical Group of Southern California
Anaheim, CA 92807
USA

JAY S. COOPER, MD
Director, Radiation Oncology
New York University Medical Center
566 First Avenue
New York, NY 10016
USA

Ralph R. Dobelbower, MD, PhD, FACR
Chairman, Department of Radiation Oncology
Medical College of Ohio
P.O. Box 10008
Toledo, OH 43699–0008
USA

Robert W. Edland, MD
Chairman, Department of Radiation Oncology
Gundersen Clinic
1836 South Avenue
La Crosse, WI 54601
USA

Anas M. El-Mahdi, MD, ScD, FACR
Department of Radiation Oncology and Biophysics
Eastern Virginia Medical School
600 Gresham Drive
Norfolk, VA 23507–1999
USA

Helmuth Goepfert, MD
Professor and Chairman, Department of Head and Neck Surgery
The University of Texas
MD Anderson Cancer Center
1515 Holcombe Blvd.
Houston, TX 77030–4095
USA

Alfred L. Goldson, MD, FACR
Chairman, Department of Radiation Therapy
Howard University Hospital
2041 Georgia Avenue, N.W.
Washington, DC 20060
USA

Thomas W. Griffin, MD
Chairman, Department of Radiation Oncology
University of Washington, Medical Center RC-08
1959 N.E. Pacific
Seattle, WA 98195
USA

S. Gupta, MD
Department of Radiation Oncology
Medical College of Ohio
P.O. Box 10008
Toledo, OH 43699–0008
USA

Edward C. Halperin, MD
Associate Professor, Division of Radiation Oncology
Duke University Medical Center
P.O. Box 3085
Durham, NC 27710
USA

J. Carlos Hernandez, MD
Assistant Professor, Department of Radiation Oncology and Nuclear Medicine
Hahnemann University
Broad and Vine Sts., Mail Stop 200
Philadelphia, PA 19102-1192
USA

David H. Hussey, MD
College of Medicine
Department of Radiology
The University of Iowa
200 Hawkins Dr., # W 1892 GH
Iowa City, IA 52242–1009
USA

Nathan Kaufman, MD
Department of Radiation Oncology
Medical College of Virginia
Virginia Commonwealth University
MCV Station, Box 58
Richmond, VA 23298–0058
USA

Herbert D. Kerman, MD
Regional Oncology Center
Halifax Medical Center
Clyde Morris Blvd.
P.O. Box 2830
Daytona Beach, FL 32115–2830
USA

Henry M. Keys, MD
RROP Regional Radiation Oncology Program
47, New Scotland Avenue
Albany, NY 12208
USA

Carl M. Mansfield, MD, ScD
Radiation Oncology and Nuclear Medicine
Thomas Jefferson University Hospital
1020 Walnut Street
Philadelphia, PA 19107–5587
USA

James E. Marks, MD
Department of Radiotherapy
Loyola University Medical Center
2160 S. First Avenue
Maywood, IL 60153
USA

Stanton A. Marks, MD
Department of Radiation Oncology
Columbia Hospital
2025 East Newport Ave.
Milwaukee, WI 53211
USA

Bizhan Micaily, MD
Department of Radiation Oncology and Nuclear Medicine
Hahnemann University
230 N. Broad St., M.S. 200
Philadelphia, PA 19102
USA

Michael J. Miller, MD
Southern California Permanente Medical Group
Radiation Oncology
4950 Sunset Blvd.
Los Angeles, CA 90027
USA

William T. Moss, MD
Department of Radiation Oncology
Oregon Health Sciences University
3181 S.W. Sam Jackson Park Road
Portland, OR 97201
USA

Kevin Murray, MD
Assistant Professor, Radiation Oncology
Medical College of Wisconsin
8700 West Wisconsin Avenue
Milwaukee, WI 53226
USA

Lester J. Peters, MD
The University of Texas
MD Anderson Cancer Center, Box 97
1515 Holcombe Blvd.
Houston, TX 77030–4095
USA

Richard D. Pezner, MD
Division of Radiation Oncology
City of Hope Medical Center
1500 E. Duarte Road
Duarte, CA 91010–0269
USA

Leonard R. Prosnitz, MD
Department of Radiation Oncology
Duke University Medical Center
Box 3085–154
Durham, NC 27710
USA

Milton Raben, MD
Department of Radiation Therapy
Bowman Gray School of Medicine
300 S. Hawthorne Road
Winston-Salem, NC 27175
USA

H. Reiter, MD
Department of Radiation Oncology
University of Rochester Medical Center
601 Elmwood Avenue, Box 647
Rochester, NY 14642
USA

Tyvin A. Rich, MD
Department of Radiotherapy
University of Texas
MD Anderson Cancer Center
1515 Holcombe Blvd.
Houston, TX 77030
USA

Philip Rubin, MD
Department of Radiation Oncology
University of Rochester Medical Center
601 Elmwood Avenue, Box 647
Rochester, NY 14642
USA

Monica Ryoo, MD
Kaiser Permanente
Southern California Permanente Medical Group
Radiation Oncology
4950 Sunset Blvd.
Los Angeles, CA 90027
USA

Robert H. Sagerman, MD
Radiation Oncology Division
SUNY Health Science Center Syracuse
750 E. Adams Street
Syracuse, NY 13210–2339
USA

Omar M. Salazar, MD
Department of Radiation Oncology
University of Maryland Medical Center
22 South Greene Street
Baltimore, MD 21201
USA

Rupert K. Schmidt-Ulrich, MD
Department of Radiation Oncology
Medical College of Virginia
Virginia Commonwealth University
MCV Station, Box 58
Richmond, VA 23298–0058
USA

Carol L. Shields, MD
Staff Surgeon, Ocular Oncology Service
Wills Eye Hospital
Assistant Professor of Ophthalmology
Thomas Jefferson University
Ninth and Walnut Sts.
Philadelphia, PA 19107
USA

Jerry A. Shields, MD
Director, Oncology Service
Wills Eye Hospital
Professor of Ophthalmology
Thomas Jefferson University
Ninth and Walnut Sts.
Philadelphia, PA 19107
USA

Burton L. Speiser, MD
Department of Radiation Oncology
St Joseph's Hospital and Medical Center
Phoenix, AZ 85013
USA

Alan D. Steinfeld, MD
Department of Radiation Oncology
New York University Medical Center
566 First Avenue
New York, NY 10016
USA

Mohan Suntharalingam, MD
Department of Radiation Oncology
University of Maryland Medical Center
22 South Greene Street
Baltimore, MD 21201
USA

Michael Tome, MD
Kaiser Permanente
Southern California Permanente Medical Group
Radiation Oncology
4950 Sunset Blvd.
Los Angeles, CA 90027
USA

Daphne Y. Tong, MD
Radiation Oncologist
Group Health Hospital
200 15th Avenue, East
Seattle, WA 98112
USA

Jonathan Tsao, MD
Kaiser Permanente
Southern California Permanente Medical Group
Radiation Oncology
4950 Sunset Blvd.
Los Angeles, CA 90027
USA

J. Frank Wilson, MD
Department of Radiation Oncology
Milwaukee County Medical Complex
Milwaukee, WI 53226
USA

Springer-Verlag and the Environment

We at Springer-Verlag firmly believe that an international science publisher has a special obligation to the environment, and our corporate policies consistently reflect this conviction.

We also expect our business partners – paper mills, printers, packaging manufacturers, etc. – to commit themselves to using environmentally friendly materials and production processes.

The paper in this book is made from low- or no-chlorine pulp and is acid free, in conformance with international standards for paper permanency.

MIX
Papier aus verantwortungsvollen Quellen
Paper from responsible sources
FSC® C105338

If you have any concerns about our products,
you can contact us on
ProductSafety@springernature.com

In case Publisher is established outside the EU,
the EU authorized representative is:
Springer Nature Customer Service Center GmbH
Europaplatz 3, 69115 Heidelberg, Germany

Printed by Libri Plureos GmbH
in Hamburg, Germany